EXERCISES THAT WORK FOR YOU

Non-strenuous fitness basics for
body, mind and spirit

Elizabeth Graham-Smith

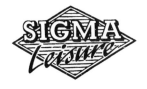

Copyright © Elizabeth Graham-Smith, 1995

All Rights Reserved. No part of this publication may be reproduced, stored in a retrieval system, or transmitted in any form or by any means – electronic, mechanical, photocopying, recording, or otherwise – without prior written permission from the publisher.

Published by Sigma Leisure – an imprint of
Sigma Press, 1 South Oak Lane, Wilmslow, Cheshire SK9 6AR, England.

British Library Cataloguing in Publication Data
A CIP record for this book is available from the British Library.

ISBN: 1-85058-431-1

Typesetting and Design by: Sigma Press, Wilmslow, Cheshire.

Cover Design and Illustrations: Design House, Marple Bridge

Printed by: MFP Design & Print

Disclaimer: Only you can judge your own suitability for any programme of exercise. If you are at all concerned about the use of any exercises in this book you should consult your own medical adviser. Neither the publisher nor the author can accept any responsibility for any injury howsoever caused as a result of the use of this book

Foreword

Those who attended her classes for the over-50s know that the young-looking teacher in the green tracksuit is a very special kind of person. Elizabeth Graham-Smith demonstrates and teaches a series of graceful movements that seem to reach joints and muscles I hardly knew I had. But more important are her warm voice and personality which are reflected in this book. She invites the reader to join in an exploration of our bodies and the range of our movements but she also finds parallel ways of exercising minds and spirits to contribute to our balance of health and self healing.

Detailed instructions enable us to follow the exercises, and her scientific background illuminates our understanding of our descent from animals and encourages a new appreciation of the way we move.

This is an up-to-date book written with the help of modern technology but its holistic approach points the way to positive thinking and an enlargement of the spirit. A special kind of manual, it will provide help for many who are trapped in today's mechanistic and commercially orientated society.

Dr Jean Coope, M.D. F.R.C.G.P.

Preface

If exercise has always felt like a boring chore for you, here is an opportunity to change that experience and perhaps your view of what an exercise is. A *real* exercise is an activity that we do purposefully, for a positive reason, taking time specially for it, and knowing exactly what it is doing for us while we are doing it. Then we go back to real life and use the results of that, and the insights and extra liveliness gained, to enrich the rest of life.

It is when we forget about the purpose and are not quite sure about the benefits either, that dissatisfaction creeps in.

Sometimes quite ordinary things that we are doing or even our present exercise programme may be working against us. If you notice that you seem to be getting shorter or your posture is developing kinks, you may even be producing those results accidentally by the way you sit or stand or even exercise. When clear about exercises that will always work for and not against us, we make a few changes for ourselves, notice definite improvements and stop being bored.

No one will turn into a glamorous superstar overnight from reading this book! It is not about glamour, nor is it a high powered training manual for sports or athletics. It is for everyday folk at any age, looking for everyday guidance for maintaining and improving their everyday fitness. But as a happy, almost incidental bonus you will feel and look much more alive if you follow these exercises, and the sports you play and all other activities will benefit too.

The core of this book is its physical exercise programme and its analysis of principles to guide our choice of exercises towards those that really work for us. But bodies, minds and spirits are involved together in our fitness and it is much more interesting to work with the full team. So there are suggestions here for supplementing physical exercise with some simple non-physical exercises to open up this broader, B/M/S front. Let mind and spirit join in! Little by little you will find you can shed the old habits that did not work for you as you introduce carefully chosen exercises that can and will.

The 20th century has been a time of huge expansion of knowledge. Human beings have been amassing more and more knowledge about the world and about the workings of bodies and minds too. Now, towards the end of the 20th century the emphasis has been changing. We still like to go on adding to the detail of all this learning but are becoming increasingly interested in the integration of all the separate specialities. Previously compartmented knowledge is finding more and more connections between the compartments within every field and between fields that used to be thought of as quite separate. We find that the whole is greater than, and increasingly more interesting, than the parts.

With this general shift of thinking to bigger contexts, attitudes to exercise are also making changes. Anticipate the 21st century! Welcome the links between body, mind and spirit. Make a few more of them! Dig those team members out of their boxes! Exercise for each of them with the whole of you in mind!

Elizabeth Graham-Smith

1

Opening Up

For exercise to make a significant difference to our fitness it should become fully integrated into our life style. We should know where we are with it. We should get to grips with why we need it and how best we can use it. It is well worthwhile to be clear about all that exercise means to us in all aspects of life.

In this introductory chapter I take a number of issues that are involved where ordinary everyday fitness is concerned, and spread them out for inspection. It is like an overture and we return to many of the themes later. If you prefer to start right in with the exercises, do return to this introduction later. You have a much higher chance of sticking to any programme if you have thought about some of these issues. These are exercises that make all the rest of life work better and we have a big advantage if we know why that is so.

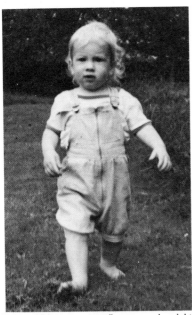 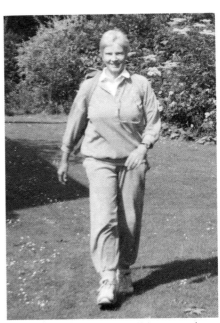

Young children are naturally open and upright. They forge straight ahead. . .   . . . adults can do the same if they remember

Facing in the Right Direction

I like to get hypochondriasis out of the way when I recommend exercising. Hypochondriacs are preoccupied with ailments and illnesses, and very often they seem doomed to a succession of further ailments and illnesses. A negative emphasis works like that. It acts to keep pulling us back. Fitness *freaking* is also unwise unless your career involves sacrificing long-term overall fitness for some short term gains. An obsessional preoccupation either with ill health or with exercising is likely to do more harm than good.

We are not hypochondriacs when we direct a sensible share of our energies towards wholesome, positive, better-than-average health. And this book chooses that practical and positive direction. It encourages body mind and spirit to work together in establishing a strong and positive forward, and upward and outward directedness.

I also like to get perfection out of the way! Wanting to be perfect is a big generator of guilt about not being so, and although a little realistic guilt can turn us to better things, too much is also among life's negatives. Somehow we need to set ourselves high standards to motivate our actions without beating ourselves up when we fall short of them.

I appreciate the work that goes into being always beautiful and always perfectly groomed and 100% fit. But I encouraged those I taught to accept and enjoy who they were and how they looked, exactly as they were – young or old, fat or thin, perfectly themselves. That then becomes the starting point for improvements to come. We expressed our individuality cheerfully, wearing comfortable track suits or leggings or shorts with T-shirts. We were main-stream non specialists, exercising for pleasure and to enrich our lives.

This book asks you to start from that acceptance too. You don't have to be perfect. You already are pretty marvellous! But you may also be interested in taking a few steps towards being even more wonderful! That is a much healthier start than looking to an idealised model, cringing with guilt at your imperfections, and then over-striving to reach an imaginary perfection. Such straining does more harm than good. We rarely stand perfectly or sit, move, behave, think, eat or relate to each other perfectly. But a picture of balanced integrity in any of these actions gives us something to return to after our unconscious lapses.

You can get good value even if you only skim the contents of this book and think about them! But you will get much more from it if you also use it seriously for its practical work and return to it for reference. When a particular member of the team in your personal body/mind/spirit outfit starts to let you know that it needs a little maintenance work, don't ask yourself: "What's wrong with me now?", (the hypochondriac's cry), but ask instead: "What is the best forward directed step I can take now?" There are plenty of guidelines and exercises here to point you to that positive and forward looking orientation.

Common Sense

I have given few references to specific research in these pages. The Bibliography and my Acknowledgements may be used as a guide to some sources and inspiration. But where *certainty* and a scientific authority are not available to support a viewpoint, I use, and ask the reader to use, some imaginative right brain talents.

When I declare, for example, that our evolution has been in a certain manner, or our brain or psychology work in this way or that, or that the human spirit has certain qualities, I ask you not to fret if the picture I give does not have documented scientific credentials or agree exactly with your own beliefs. It is sometimes just a picture! We can use the remarkably valuable gift of human imagination, and our personal images, very creatively to keep making a positive difference to our health.

I trained in and respect objective scientific disciplines and I do not deliberately paint false pictures. But as in many other areas of enquiry today, movement and exercise are due for a much more broad fronted, right-brain inclusive approach. The time has come to look at the needs of our body/mind/spirit holistically and imaginatively, and this is what I do. Our ordinary common sense can embrace a wide acceptance, both of the wonders science has brought to us and any inner enrichment our creative imagination can contribute.

Taking Exercise is Special: Commitment to Positive Change

I always recognised something special about the people who came to my classes, and that specialness is there for all who take exercise purposefully. Taking exercise, after all, simply means doing something active (instead of just wishing), in order to change or improve something we want to change or improve. There is a commitment made by any person who chooses to do something positive for a personal goal or purpose. I believe this commitment to positive change to be a natural driving mechanism for humans. I would like to help to keep it alive for people who already have it, and help to generate it anew if this or any other self help work is new to you.

How Should We Choose an Exercise for the Body?

Exercises for the body have come a long way since people first thought about exercising. Some of the earliest were invented for soldiers and athletes needing tough and specialised training. I can still remember the gym mistress's fierce commands when I was at school, and the pressure of her knee in the small of my back even at school dinners. That was the style for many of my generation, at school in the 1930s and '40s. Fortunately, I also remember glowing with pleasure when she said I was like a monkey on the bars and ropes in the gym. That positive right brain picture probably made a much bigger difference to my pleasure in gymnastics, athletics and sport than did her sergeant-major shouting or her knee in my back.

Today we are more conscious of natural movements, and we know that most children and adults are not in need of a military, highly regimented fitness programme and could be damaged by it. We do need some discipline, and sufficiently intelligent exercise to enable us to stay limber and balanced and handle our lives optimally, and we need enough reserve in our fitness to be able to meet a sudden emergency. We do not, for everyday well-being need undue stresses and masochism. We do need good pictures and visions. Our personal inner pictures of how we would like ourselves to be, and what we like to see in the fitness of other people are both very valuable guides. Very few of us really admire slouching and sloppiness!

Natural Movement and Mechanical Good Sense, too

Chapters 2 and 3 present guidelines that can help us to make up for the natural movements missing from modern lives. We should keep an eye, for example, on the big range of movements that developing human bodies have used for thousands of years and let it guide some of our own.

Then we also need to watch the way in which we use the engineering of the structure we inherit, so that we do not make the mistake of putting ours at risk. Today's world is a very different one from that of our ancestors. While Chapter 2 explores some of the evolved expectations of bodies, Chapter 3 pin-points, in a much simplified way, some of the main engineering considerations that should also guide us.

There used to be a popular exercise called *jumping jacks* or *star jumps*. People still use it. If we are very light and limber it is perfectly safe. But it is much more likely, since the average human being is comparatively stiff and often overweight today, that it will stress our under-exercised joints and jar our more rigid spine. Imagine a polar bear or a monkey keeping fit with star jumps!

Our ancestors the apes, would never force their arms and legs to stretch hard in two opposite directions at once, for one fruit on one side, say, and another from the opposite

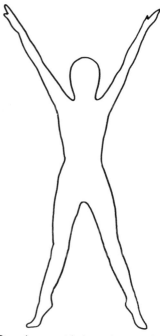

Strongly symmetrical exercises may jar the framework

side, jumping up and down as they did so! Their *exercise* would be the smooth natural movement of reaching one way and then another simply to satisfy a need. Gentle stretches of this sort are right for us, too. No engineer would inflict long periods of those pounding movements without strengthening the joints to handle such a beating and making sure that the whole framework could take that prolonged jarring. We should keep an eye on the mechanical risks when we use movements that are clearly unnatural.

"One limb at a time, and lightly", is more natural, and therefore a sounder approach to most exercises than rigidly symmetrical or jerky snatch-and-grab movements. Watch a forest bear as it clambers over trees and rocks. Even the trapeze artist, like the ape, reaches for the bar with a smooth one/two arrival. Most of the exercises I recommend avoid any unnaturally symmetrical use of the limbs.

Throughout the animal kingdom we can watch the graceful flow of movement. Not just in the apes, our immediate ancestors, but from amoeba to centipede, and in young children too where they have been allowed a free range of movement as infants; there is an air of exploring rather than grabbing at life with their movements.

We see the same easy grace in acrobatic movement, and in many traditional dances or the gentle martial art of Tai Chi. Grace has succeeded biologically, socially and even in skilled hand-to-hand fighting. It is built into us to enjoy both making and watching movements that are both soft and fluid and

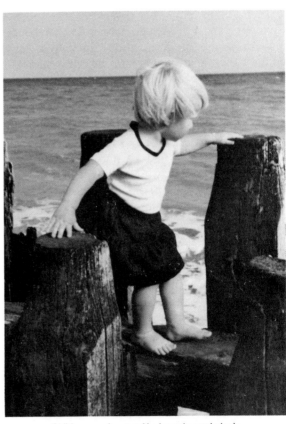

Children reach out softly, bravely, exploringly

mechanically sound. We find them beautiful. Stretching exercises, even in our fitness programme, should have the same smooth and unforced quality and large expansiveness of the graceful yawns and stretches we make when we are waking up.

Not only does your body not want to be jarred, it takes time to recover from jarring. The early exercise pioneers who introduced physical jerks should not be blamed for ignorance. They only overdid movements of this sort out of a genuine awakening enthusiasm for any movement at all, with perhaps just a little military aggressiveness and self punishment there too. Basically their reasons were good because a growing fitness problem has been recognised as civilisation has changed the patterns of human life. But today we need a different sort of enthusiasm: much less regimentation and a kinder, more user-friendly and holistic approach to exercise.

We can probably never compensate ourselves fully for the loss of those exuberant patterns of movement from the long ages of evolutionary history. Our genes may still yearn to swing in trees and race across plains. I am sure my body misses these challenging, wide ranging activities with some deep inner longing. A walk down the lane sometimes seems a very poor substitute.

By the time we leave school we have already stopped using the uninhibited movements that we enjoyed as children. We used to leap and roll and stretch and swing ourselves around. But one day our mothers and teachers began to complain that we should be "more grown up now". We stopped spreading our legs or flinging our arms quite so widely, and the gradual shutting down and closing off began. Culture and civilisation claimed us. They began to exert their subtle and continuous pressures. We cut back with one small inhibition after another and have gradually reduced the wonderful range and variety of everyday movements that is really natural to us.

Knowing that this is one of life's hazards, we can choose to reverse that process. If we want to claim back suppleness and good posture and enjoy freely flowing movement again we need to exercise every joint and muscle gently and regularly. We probably need an exercise supplement more than we need any nutritional supplements. Joints need to be loosened where stiff, and muscles need to be lightly stretched and encouraged to release unnecessary tensions, not once in a lifetime but regularly and frequently.

And quite apart from any specific programme of exercises, we should give ourselves freedom to play more, to be adventurous and to release the child in us in many ways. Active fun and lively play are very good exercises.

Don't Forget the Brain

Minds as well as bodies carry a huge backlog of memories and conditioning. For minds, this laying down of patterns has not come from specific genetic rules but from a more generalised ability to adapt that the genes provide. Your mind and its idiosyncrasies are uniquely yours. They grew up in intimate association with your body, shaped by your personal history and culture and events around you.

So brains, although part of our evolved make-up, are probably even more individual than are human bodies, and minds often become stuck in fairly strong patterns of behaviour, conditioned by events in our lives. We have been *designing* our personal patterns of nerve networks all along to handle the specific experiences that have come our way. Shocks have sometimes para-lysed neural pathways. But changes and new pathways can always be made, even if we have no idea how that can possibly happen physically in the nerve networks themselves.

We do not have to be psychologists or neurologists to get a glimpse of some of the ways in which our mind and brain work, but we do have to detach ourselves a little to think about them at all. If we have an imaginative sympathy with the mind's limitations as well as its possibilities and ways in which it might operate, this can illuminate the whole body/mind relationship.

Human beings have an interesting left-brain/right-brain differentiation that is becoming increasingly familiar to us today. Again, we only need an approximate picture to use. Bi-pedalism was a major change as humans became more distinctively human. Language and thinking, creating tribes, agriculture, culture and tools, were all happening at the same time. Changes in all these developments at once have taken the human animal into very new directions, nerve networks and needs. The emerging human took over the quadruped's brain and began to put the adaptable possibilities of the two hemispheres to different tasks in different ways.

Table 1 lists some of the divisions of labour that we now associate with the two partially distinct sides of the brain. Many factors in that differentiation can affect our use of exercise. Coordination exercises are especially valuable in helping to further cooperation between the two sides when they seem to be in opposition, and even help to integrate the two sides of our human nature. The table may not apply to absolutely everybody in every detail but it is a well accepted generalisation. Even advertisers use these categories to reach and influence us.

In our quadruped ancestors, the *wiring* of the two brain hemispheres was such that each side managed the movement for the opposite side of the body. We still have that arrangement and I shall often refer to it. But when the development of language needed newly specialised brain skills it was the left hemisphere that adapted to this need. On this left side the big difference is in the skills of handling information linearly, processing one event at a time. Words, letters and numbers have to be used one at a time, and the tasks of logic, calculation, reading and writing are all managed here, step by step.

Table 1

The left brain manages	The right brain manages
Right side of the body	Left side of the body
Writing and numbers	Creative ideas
Time and timetables	Space and movement
Analysis	Putting things together
Reasoning	Music
Being objective	Grasping whole concepts
First steps in learning	Integrating new information
Trying too hard	Letting ideas come
Detailed examination	Seeing the whole picture

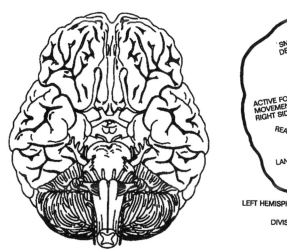 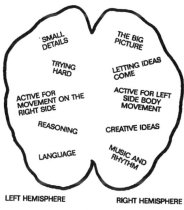

Division of labour in the brain

The left brain skills are somewhat like those of a computer, though today's machines can now calculate much faster than we can. We can be well organised and efficient if the left brain takes good charge of our activities. Its logical expertise has been an extremely important development for humans.

The right side of the brain works for us in a more intuitive and creative and all-embracing way. The skills here are older ones, taking in and integrating information on a wide front all at once, as wild animals must. Free and well coordinated movement is one of these basics, so is the subtle grasp of pre-language sounds, and the enjoyment of music which originated in those ancient sounds. Our flashes of creative insights and ecstasies and visions all happen here on this right side.

The difference in these right and left brain skills is rather like the difference between peripheral and narrowly focused vision. Both can and should operate at once. But sometimes one side of the brain seems to dominate our actions and choices. The right will often ignore some sensible and logical promptings from the left. Or the left may dominate and close itself off from the creativity or wild schemes of the right side and feel very *right*, critical and judgmental about those.

It is the more tender, less *hard wired* right hemisphere side of our intelligence that often suffers from today's strong emphasis on high technology and regimentation of skills. A too analytical and left brain approach can hamper human creativity. Thoughts and feelings from creative right brain activity can be quite difficult to express in words just because of this all-at-once mode of operation. The right side was very accomplished in its own way long before speech developed, and we cannot analyse its talents. We have to use them intuitively without trying too hard to pin them down.

Scientific geniuses probably work with the logic and intuition of left and right sides operating in full cooperation. Poets and artists and musicians have to find their own ways around the problem of expressing subtle right brain feelings. They have to coax *linear* ways of expressing themselves. Many art forms have developed as humans have wanted to share this broader elusive right brain experience. When we are attracted to an artist's, musician's or dancer's work, our right brain is probably responding intuitively to the right brain perception they were expressing via their chosen left-brain, one-step-at-a-time notation or brush strokes. Similarly, when we act as music or art critics, or wine tasters, for example, we have to use imaginative and evocative expressions as metaphors if we want to sum up our impressions and speak or write about those hard to analyse works of art.

Learning Needs Both Sides of the Brain

We need both sides of the brain when we set out to explore anything new, from a new language to a new commitment to exercise! While the left brain busies itself with rules and principles, the right side will be doing a behind-the-scenes job of integrating and assessing and taking on board the information it intuitively recognises as valuable. It will be making subtle choices. It is an important partner.

Later, the right brain may take in completely the poem or song or the subtleties of holding the cricket bat or riding a bicycle that it has struggled with, and be able to reproduce it almost automatically. Like rope sight for bell ringers it can happen in a sudden flash of insight.

For this partnership of learning to work best, we have to occupy the left brain with some well structured plans. We give it work to do of the kind it is happy with, which will also keep it from being too judgmental! And we have to liberate the right by not being too serious in our approach. Our right brain backs away if the left dominates too strongly and shouts its criticisms and "no's". We need to use every trick we can think of to relax the right hemisphere and encourage its cooperation.

Right brain cooperation as it relates to healthy exercise is encouraged by keeping the programme cheerful and unregimented. There is no fun in parade ground drills. Then, because the right brain loves positive and beautiful pictures, it also helps to have a clear and lovely vision of the new liveliness and fitness towards which we are working. Your right brain welcomes and thrives on such positive visionary input, especially if you are doing something towards it and not just hoping or wishing.

We benefit in all areas of our life from taking a little trouble to create *right-brain-friendly* surroundings. Music and flowers and colour and landscape and relaxed human company are all right-brain stimulants. If we provide ourselves with these they help us to stay balanced in today's world of straight lines and machinery and high computerised technology.

A very high-tech style of interior design can subtly hamper our personal creativity, our learning and even our general well-being. To balance school or office situations, people instinctively soften a harsh environment with plants and flowers and escape into the countryside for holidays and at weekends. If you enjoy listening to opera, you have probably felt that the exuberant decoration of the opera house makes a real contribution to the musical experience. Striped wallpaper would not be the same! Warmly beautiful surroundings relax the right brain which then becomes more open and receptive to the music. When our right brain is looked after, the benefits of balancing left and right sides will gradually filter through to enrich all aspects of our life.

If you exercise at home, try working in the garden sometimes, or with a view of trees and landscape, or at least have something real nearby such as flowers on a window sill or just a beautiful picture. If you have to exercise in a high-tech gym, make sure to laugh and play and brighten your environment with colourful clothes. Avoid synthesised or harsh music, or music with a very strong marching beat. Coax the right brain and you will find an enthusiasm and vision that lasts longer than any effort produced by trying to coerce or bully yourself.

Coordination Across the Hemispheres

Because we are bipeds using a quadrupedally evolved structure, our physical coordination uses a crisscross of nerve connections across brain and body, and spiralling muscle linkages across and around the body. Eyesight has even more complex brain linkages. Each eye has both right and left brain connections before their nerves converge at the central visual cortex at the back of the brain. We should stay wide awake visually all the time we exercise, keeping all these optical linkages active, too. Let your eyes enjoy both the detail of shapes of objects and the broad sweep of your surroundings.

We tax that physical crisscross coordination lightly in this programme and keep the nerve networks active with the very simple *cross-crawl* exercises. Through improving those physical linkages they become energisers for the whole team of body, mind and spirit.

Relaxation, Suppleness, and Getting Muscle Tone Right

It is vitally important to our fitness, and a major theme in this book, to release excess tension. We really have to keep at it! Unwanted tensions anywhere are the negatives that filter through into the workings of body, brain, mind, spirit and emotions, too. Try tensing your seat muscles now, and notice what happens to your breathing as that tension travels round the body.

Techniques for physical tension release include both non-stressed movement and bodily rest, through aware exercise and specific periods of relaxation. But we can also let go via painting imaginary pictures in mental exercises, by letting old emotional hang-ups go, and in choosing positive tonics for our minds and spiritual lives. All these activities belong in a fitness programme for the whole person.

Not all tension is harmful, of course. There is a *just right* balance between letting all muscle power go, and retaining enough to stay active and poised for the tasks in hand. In some emergencies we may need extreme tension to extricate ourselves from danger. Obviously, without some muscular effort our skeleton couldn't possibly hold itself up. We use the word *tone* for this necessary amount of tension and we like it to be appropriate to a particular situation. It has its counterpart in mental and perhaps even the spiritual strength we are using at any time, and its level will vary. If we remain unaware of our choice in the matter, the body tone we adopt may be dictated by habit alone and this is unwise. We then bring too little strength to some tasks, or too much to others, instead of exactly what is needed.

If you opt for a life spent mostly in an armchair, and a do-it-for-me approach, make sure you can continue to afford the help of others to prop you up in old age. Both the sofa habit and a reluctance to act autonomously lead to low muscle tone. If we think of a scale of 10, an addiction to armchairs can lead to almost zero tone and carry quite a health risk. When we are normally active and relaxed and not over-stressed, healthy muscle tone will be somewhere in the middle of this hypothetical scale. When very pushed in a high powered and stressful job, we should be able to increase our muscle tone to 9 or 10 appropriately, and reduce it again between bouts of stressful activity.

Deliberately toning the muscles through exercise shows us the value of a well toned body, so that, having both exercised and thought about it, we can then save the extremes of limpness and martial rigidity for extreme occasions, or leave them right behind us until we die.

Is the Pursuit of Fitness Selfish?

Some of us may look on personal exercise and possibly other self-improvement work as very selfish and unproductive. It sometimes seems so. I expect that even saints occasionally wonder if they are devoting too much time to their spiritual well-being! But dismissing exercises as selfish stops short of the true situation. Everything in the living universe thrives on care and attention, as our friendships, family and pets, gardens, clothes, houses, cars, environment and all of civilisation demonstrates. We should not leave ourselves out of that picture. We thrive on care and attention, too.

It is an illusion that we are caring better for others when we leave ourselves out. Self care is only ultimately selfish if it is a complete preoccupation. In fact we are much better at caring of any sort when we keep ourselves physically, mentally and spiritually fit, and operate from a secure level of self cherishing. What you do for yourself, to enhance bodily, mental or spiritual fitness has its spin-off value in everything you do for others.

It is probably much more selfish to withdraw our fitness from friends and family, and this is what we are doing when neglecting our own health. We then inevitably make more and more demands upon others. Looking after our own fitness in positive ways is a major responsibility to ourselves, and one of the biggest contributions we can make to society.

Positive Motivation

Negative motivation is much too often our trigger when we decide to follow a particular course. We buy a book on exercises or join a class because we think we are starting to look old and bent, or because we want to avoid pain and disability. We easily slip into this trap and, of course, advertisers know this habit well and can often sell to us because of our fears and anxieties.

But this book is all about reversing that direction of thinking. My recommendation is that we bring a totally, even extravagantly positive approach to our personal exercise programme. In body, mind, spirit and imagination we actually need all the plus we can muster! When we tackle exercise from a negative point of view the result will almost always be a neglecting of the book or a giving up of the project. To get away from this trap of accumulating one negative after another it is an exercise in itself to exaggerate its opposite and go right over the top in a bold about-face.

So try this positive exercise! First of all drop all inner and outer hesitations and grumbles or guilts about fitness or your shortcomings or anything else! (Big Job!) Especially drop the *minus-speak* that gives a non-stop negative commentary on life, people, the government, your health, the future of your country, humanity, everything! Then instead of thinking and speaking about exercises as a way of not becoming a conspicuously poor specimen of a degenerate and doomed human race, turn all those negatives on their head. Decide that you bought or borrowed this book because you intend to become, not *perfect* – there is no such thing, remember, but a super specimen of this fantastically promising species! This creative shift of viewpoint will bring positive and lasting results as well as being an amusing exercise.

You will not just be facing in a better direction, you will start to take positive steps in that direction. Exercise itself will acquire a forward looking positive aspect, an invitation to better things.

Positive Means Generous Creative and Optimistic

When we look back negatively, and only concentrate on a past full of our illnesses and accidents, say, or focus in the present on unwanted stiffness, or look gloomily forwards as if towards a future that we mistrust and dread, we are simply emphasising just one side of the huge range of possibilities in those assorted life situations and time zones. In fact, anything can happen, and that which has happened is neutralised already, just by being over. We can train ourselves imaginatively to be creatively generous in thought and words towards all these time frames, past present and future, not just to our own health and self esteem and towards other people.

Optimism is a kind of generosity. It needs the same conscious effort that all other creative activities need, but it is a directional skill well worth acquiring.

Make a point of noticing even the tiniest of positive results from the simplest of your exercises. Even "That felt good!", will face you in a better direction and will start to shift your fitness along in the direction of plus that we all need.

Body/Mind and Spirit: The Linkages

There is continuous traffic between minds and bodies, so much so that our body/mind is generally recognised to be a composite entity. Nerves and blood vessels are bringing signals to cells and organs all the time. But sometimes a physical response is not totally released. If we have a huge injury, for example, or even stay feeling hurt after a minor one, either physical or mental, or if our mind misinterprets a signal and *takes offence* or overacts in self defence, muscles can tighten too much and fail to release all the tension used. Then the chemistry of the body goes wrong. We can imagine toxins locked up in the nerve networks and in the muscles.

Unresolved fears and emotions and negative attitudes all lead to habits of physical tension and these steadily reduce the chemical and hormonal efficiency that bodies properly expect to have. Even our immunity to disease can suffer in this interactive body/mind process.

We can learn to become much more watchful of our mental attitudes. We can actually choose to cultivate more positive ones. It is not just a vague influence that thoughts and statements are having. They are penetrating our nerves and muscles and doing active harm or good, steadily undermining or topping us up all the time. When aware of this we have a choice. I would rather choose to top up my body chemistry than run it down.

Try the awareness technique of exaggerating a habit or an action when you want to see its effects more clearly. We can do this bodily, or with any of our habits of *minus-speak* or other negative mental patterns and simply see what happens.

One useful exaggeration is to imagine that our mental attitudes actually are our immune system, and that they alone and nothing else are organising the body/mind to stay healthy and well. This is not the whole picture, of course, but by thinking in this overkill way, about the big influence our words and thoughts and attitudes undoubtedly have, we can start to take those things more seriously. We can then incorporate more of those deliberately chosen positive attitudes, actions and words more often into our way of living.

The interface between the body/mind entity and our human spirit is not so easy to describe. No scientists in white overalls have measured blood pressure, heart rate, hormones etc. to correlate with spiritual activities. It may also work via the same electrical and chemical processes of nerves and hormones, but my right brain prefers to see this spirit connection as sheer magic!

We need a right-brain image for the human spirit, an expansive one that can roam between and outside all the chemical and physical processes of the world, and inside each one of us too. The big abstract word spirit is limitless. I use "human spirit" in this book, for the subtle human quality that intuitively takes our own personal body/mind into relationship with other people and links us to the rest of the universe around us. It extends beyond our body/mind. We can open our own spirit to be part of as big and as positive a spiritual abstraction or energy source as we can imagine.

Spirits are not limited by genes, history or chemistry in any way. Choose to have a very plus spirit! Let it be a *higher self* in your team, with power to guide and advise you and to cross gaps and create positive happenings. As well as noticing an interface between your spirit and body/mind, see it as interfacing, too, between you and all other people.

All the positive interactions between human beings can be viewed as spiritual as well as bodily and mental transactions once we have invented, adopted or just accepted a spiritual dimension, and they all act positively on our health and well-being as individuals. The simple, perhaps naive *spiritual exercises* of Chapter 5 are chiefly drawing attention to the bigger fitness value of making these positive links between human beings. They offer suggestions for strengthening them in down-to-earth and beneficial ways.

A Gentle Caution

Do not expect instant all-over transformation when you exercise! It is important to know that improvement is going on and to acknowledge every tiny bit, but it is also essential to allow progress to be quite slow. Gradually you will lose old restrictions and tensions and acquire, instead, new ways of expressing that vitality out into the wide world.

There is nothing in this programme that can hurt you at any age if you have ordinary average fitness and never work to a level of pain. Warm clothing and warming up exercises help muscles to release. These are especially essential to make stretching safe. Forcing a stretch in either a cold or a contracted muscle that can tear muscle fibres is the biggest hazard to watch out for if you are very unexercised and start without care. Pain tells us clearly when to stop and its messages must be respected. Be content to regain flexibility slowly, safely and surely in this way.

The exercises are all for all ages. But if you are starting the programme very late in life, smaller, almost token movements are the way to begin, leaving out any that seem difficult. Go for steadily improving mobility and alignment, not for the glamour image of the celebrity video or the total suppleness of infants and acrobats. Aim for a fitter you. If you persist with the regular loosening up and the gentlest of stretches you will soon notice a real difference that benefits you in all your actions and invites you to enjoy much more activity.

If you feel at all concerned about starting to exercise for any reason, consult your own medical adviser and take his or her advice. They might wish you to make small modifications related to your condition. But as for the spiritual exercises, they are totally without risk!

2

Guide Lines from The Past

What Does Evolution Tell Us? What DO Bodies Expect?

There are certain characteristics of animal life that we all share and most of us think little about. They may seem too obvious to be worth considering. Yet the way in which we choose to exercise can be given a new emphasis if we consider them one by one, and take each into account. Think about each one with left brain logic, and integrate them into a whole guiding pattern with your intuitive right brain.

(i) Uniqueness

We belong firmly in the animal world with all its diversity yet each of us is very special in it. In evolution's dazzling pageant, every living organism is right at the top of an unbroken line to the beginning of life, and that is a very important place to be. This does not mean it was planned that way but, nevertheless, you are right up front in it, ahead of millions of animals and humans who preceded you.

So there is no blue-print of perfection for any animal or for us, just many changing bodies and a continually shifting picture. There is no one exactly like oneself, and we have no need to imitate others though we are free to do so and sometimes benefit a lot if we use good models when we do. Each of us, within certain species and personal and community constraints, can choose our own ways of self expression.

Uniqueness has been successful in the evolutionary scheme so don't be afraid to be special or a little bit different. As long as we respect each other, our uniqueness is good for the individual, good for society and good for the human race. We are all the same but each a little bit different. We can be experimental; we can initiate actions and make changes if we want to. Keep your uniqueness in mind when choosing exercises. You are definitely special!

(ii) Movement is Vital

Every body needs to move freely. Once the earliest animal organism discovered free movement it did not go back. There was not just survival value here, but huge potential. Not that *potential* meant anything in that chance-led process. Only when those survival benefits had led to consciousness would any animal see itself as having potential.

The special pleasure that we feel in free body movement is perhaps Nature's way of ensuring we keep this essential skill, and ourselves, alive. Human bodies have evolved with a great deal of movement and plenty of space to move in and enjoy. They are now programmed to be active and to explore.

Most cultures have ways of celebrating pleasure in movement, sometimes in games or traditional dances. One of the simplest treats you can give your body is to move it around a little more and perhaps a little more freely and adventurously. Even when still, we can sometimes sense an inner movement, from all the lively systems cooperating actively inside us.

One simple recipe for a long and healthy life is to make sure we keep plenty of lively activity in it. Bus conductors, in one early research investigation, were found to live longer than bus drivers, their more active life being healthier than the sedentary one of just driving. Another long-lived breed is the musical conductor, again physically active and very expressively alive. And my guess is that window cleaners are probably more generally fit than computer buffs.

If you never, ever do an exercise, do remember to include plentiful movement in the category of vital ingredients of your life that your body is programmed to expect.

(iii) Excess Tension is Harmful. Find Ways to Release It

Animal bodies instinctively use just enough muscle tension when they move, and they release excess tension afterwards. But that no longer happens automatically in the human animal. Psychology has crept in! Our consciousness has interfered with many of the older processes. We are more clever now and more devious too. We can adopt a *stiff upper lip*, a *bold front* or a *poker face* and many other concealing or defensive patterns all involving tension, almost as a way of life. Then necks, jaws and hands grow tight, muscles shorten and joints stiffen. Every restriction absorbs a little energy and holds us back. The whole body wants to be free at any time to articulate well and as one.

If we think what happens to the skeleton of a body with unevenly tight muscles we can see it pulled down by the strain. Joints will be under compression instead of open and free. Any little bit of distortion will upset the body's alignment. A small stiffness in one area leads to another place compensating with a different tension. If we could release our local tightnesses automatically, as animals do, we might never need any exercises or become bowed down in old age. But the pressures of our human culture do make it likely that we shall always need to put in some work in this area. Consciousness and intelligence both help us to release our holding on habits.

Fortunately, there are things we can do. Even though tension may have both physical and psychological origins, a good exercise programme, regular rest and relaxation can help to release either variety. Loosening stiff joints and gently stretching muscles can even help to release deep seated anxieties and long ago fears that were part of the anchoring and armouring tension patterns taking a hold.

(iv) Human Bi-Pedalism is Very Special

The evolution of man has been one of life's most interesting experiments. No longer thought of as a planned progression, it has yet been a most extraordinary adventure. We have come a long way! We have evolved from many early ways of moving, and now we balance and walk upright on two legs. That is an enormous achievement for a process that started its experiments with a single cell. The apparently precarious balance, high above our two legs, brings huge advantages to the human animal.

But the two-sided symmetry is not an exact one. Both posture and locomotion for humans involve a balanced partnership across two not quite perfectly matched sides. It is a partnership that could be a model for all other partnerships, whether between non identical people or even races or nations. If we try to impose a very mechanical symmetry on our walking or habitually twist or jar one side strongly against the other, we set up strains in the partnership. There is scope for a little freedom for each side as well as full cooperation and mutual support.

When we do use both sides fluidly, we are almost two persons in one. We

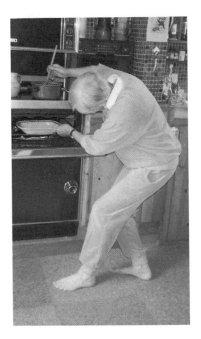
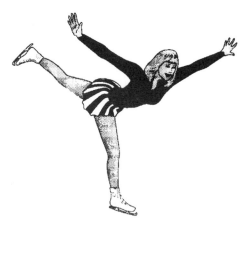

The human bi-ped is free to use each limb differently

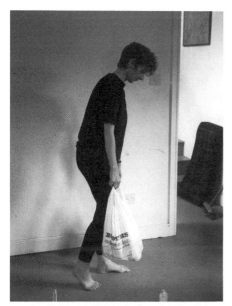
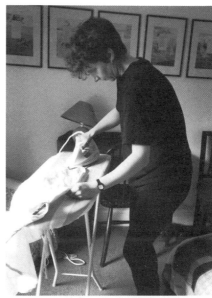
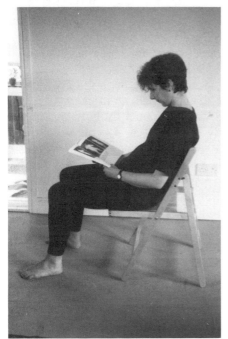
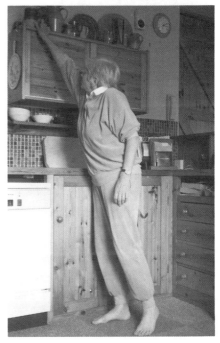

Modern life invites a variety of rather poor postures

can stir a saucepan with one hand while opening the oven door with the other. We can move with much greater freedom than any of our quadruped cousins. We can reverse, move sideways and rotate on a vertical axis, and much more. Human beings can be inventive in movement and do extraordinary things, but we should always use our bi-pedal freedom sympathetically.

(v) Uprightness is Humanity's Supreme Quality

Human uprightness, part of that bi-pedal development, is another of evolution's very clever achievements. Our ancestors, emerging from the quadrupedal limitations, discovered its value first posturally, possibly from standing on branches to reach, eat more efficiently or see further. Or perhaps in a semi-aquatic period they walked in shallow seas that supported them. Later they exploited the advantages of uprightness for racing across the plains and hunting. It has become a hall mark of humanity.

This growth towards a vertical stance has involved the slow perfection of an anti-gravity system of muscle support. Nature is inevitably surrounded by the physical laws of the universe. All of life evolved within them. She has to contend with the strong pull of gravity because the universe is held together by this force. She might seem to be constrained to limit all the life form experiments to fish supported by sea-water or slugs and serpents slithering along on land. There had to be some very clever muscular and skeletal arrangements to lift bodies off the ground at all, and these have adjusted themselves little by little over millions of years.

We have no direct conscious control over our ancient anti-gravity system, and yet it still works well and there are things we can do to keep it in good working order. We do not have to be weighed down by gravity. Animal springiness and suppleness have already developed as a response to it and operate well within it. The human body expects us to stay well aligned, and in return for good alignment it maintains its anti-gravity springiness for us. Today, maintaining a true uprightness may need a little of our conscious intervention to make up for the very different way of life humans now have. If we value uprightness we may need to think about it and work a little to retain it.

A good exercise programme is very valuable to our alignment and posture. It develops the body awareness that we need to get the most out of our inheritance of the anti-gravity muscle system and retain it for life.

A modern, complex and largely sedentary life invites a great variety of distorted postures. If we are depressed, for example, we often allow the force of gravity to slump and shorten us. If we are desk bound we may sink or slump into the chair. But habitual slumps, twists or leaning inevitably result in a gradual loss of mobility in joints, premature ageing of muscles and hardening

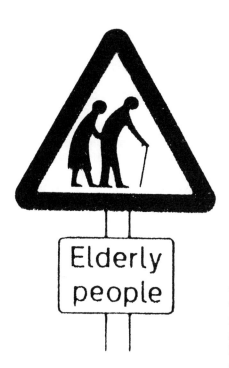

Perhaps we can avoid succumbing to gravity in this way

of connective tissues. Lungs, heart, gut, eyes, larynx and much else then have to put up with unnaturally cramped conditions and they all start to work below par. Once this process is started, simply in an unconscious habit pattern, we shall need a conscious effort to undo its effects and rescue the uprightness natural for our species.

We can obviously stay better aligned when we are supple than when stiff. The growing stiffness of ankles, backs and necks, mostly from underuse, fixes our assorted misalignments. We should keep one eye on staying nicely extended between earth and sky (largely a mental exercise), and then exercise muscles and joints to retain easy flexibility. Straining towards a rigidly vertical line, only puts in more of the unwanted tensions. Chapter 4 has more to say about this desirable alignment.

The very word *upright* is used for more than mere body alignment. We use it almost synonymously with integrity. It describes one of the qualities we most admire in human beings in an almost spiritual way. We rightly demand integrity in our leaders, and we value it in all our relationships. If we value the human experiment at all we value this special quality that it has produced. The body has its own physical integrity in uprightness, but through it we subtly sense an integrity of the individual as a whole, of mind and spirit too.

It is a positive help to our own supple physical vertical alignment if we also consciously admire this quality in others.

(vi) Length and Width are Important Dimensions

The shape of the human torso is unique in the animal world. While experimenting with uprightness, two-leggedness and manual dexterity, our ancestors gradually adjusted the distribution of their weight to gain stability higher off

the ground. The torso widened across the upper chest and became comparatively narrow in depth, so that now our back and front have roughly similar
lengths and widths. If we think only of our upright length, vital as this is, we
may lose out on this valuable across-the-body width.

A quick comparison with the torso of a fish, cow or greyhound will show
how far we have come in this adaptation away from depth and towards breadth.
The human torso shape is more like that of a playing card balanced on feet at
right angles, but without that rigidity. Both the shoulder and pelvic girdles
have opened out like the pages of a book. Width clearly has psychological
significance too because clothes fashions have often widened the shoulder line
with extra padding. Power, as well as integrity are projected then as images to
influence others by the way we dress up and present ourselves to them.

But unlike those other quadruped mammals we are able to distort the
relationship between front and back. We can fold in from side to side, or
forwards and down, rounding the shoulders, collapsing the ribs, slackening
the abdominal sheath and narrowing and shortening the front. Our four-legged
forebears could not slump if they tried! The newly vertical human spine is able
to collapse, shorten and twist, and, unfortunately, it can do these things
unawarely.

If we settle into an habitual imbalance between front and back areas, from
stooping down, rounding in or arching back unduly, we upset the way the
upright spine carries the body's weight. Muscular energy has to be used in
these distortions and this is wasteful. It leads to fatigue and, of course, by
crowding the heart, lungs, gut and the many organs needing, and expecting to
be provided with plenty of space, it hampers their action. We then operate
below par and fatigue can become chronic.

Again, human openness, like uprightness, has special value as a quality we
instinctively trust. We like to be with people who are open. We feel that they
are fully present and open to us. These two qualities go together. We need
them ourselves in body, mind and spirit and welcome them in other people.
Unstrained length and width should be honoured and given their place in every
exercise programme.

(vii) Spines are Naturally Lithe

The human spine may seem like a tent pole but it evolved to be willowy and
strong with a few light curves. It has a natural ability to maintain its strong and
supple length. It tapers and the bones are lighter towards the top. It rises
flexibly out of the pelvis and carries the weight of the head balanced on the
top vertebrae in a way that is new in the animal kingdom.

We do not have to inform ourselves of every detail of our evolution as we look for guidelines for using the spine well, but a broad pictures can be very useful. The human spine probably developed its curves in three major stages:

❏ First as our vertebrate fishy ancestors emerged from the sea with a long straight skeleton and needed a new way of looking around them

❏ Secondly in shifting from reptilian to mammalian locomotion, a little higher off the ground

❏ Finally to make possible a versatile upright human stance and walk.

The infant spine also goes through those stages, acquiring the last curves as it adjusts to an upright walk.

Now those curves – cervical, dorsal and lumbar – are still useful for resilience and shock absorption. If the human spine had not acquired curves in that process – like a vertical fish! – or if we try to straighten them out ourselves by tucking in the pelvis or the chin, we would be less able to absorb the shocks of movement. However, if we exaggerate the curves, and over-arch the back or tilt our head back or thrust it forward, we make disruptive breaks in this line which can bring problems.

Each spinal vertebra has a strong cylindrical building block as its core, and small bits sticking out of it that help it to locate and move with its neighbours. We need to carry our weight mostly through that main column and not its protuberances and protective fail-safe ligaments. Exaggerated curves will make that support column more precarious.

Then there are cushioning discs between the vertebrae, acting as buffers and giving us a springy flexibility. If you watch a great ape leap from tree to tree, it draws back first, as if shrinking before leaping, and then extends into greatly expanded length. The ape has more scope than we do, perhaps, but we do this ourselves, less obviously, when diving or even just standing up from sitting, extending all the way along the spine.

No adult has the same spinal flexibility as ape or infant, though dancers and acrobats with very specialised training, retain amazing suppleness. But we can exercise the spine to retain the suppleness we need. Our anti-gravity muscles need our flexibility all the time for their task of holding all the vertebrae lightly in optimum alignment.

(viii) Pride of Bearing/Poise is Natural

Poise is a natural quality. It takes uprightness one step further than a mere balancing act. Human bodies, just like those of other animals, are endowed by Nature with total self respect and pride in the way they carry themselves. We like to see this quality, and, as we shall often observe, that which we like to see can guide and instruct us. We admire poise in young children and in actors, dancers and statesmen, and should not feel self conscious about expressing it ourselves. Excessive modesty and self-negating habits are not good for the human animal. They compress spines and carry minds and spirits down with them, too. They even depress the people we are with.

In the animal world we rarely see unpoised postures. If there at all they are temporary patterns, used in a few submissive or aggressive behaviours, and then abandoned. But we see these exaggerations all too often in the human animal. Adults can hold on to permanently shy postures, or sometimes inflated or domineering ones, quite subconsciously, long after any initial need for such deference or aggression. It is much healthier to remember the birthright of poise with awareness and recognition, and to allow it to return to us. This may require a conscious effort and we may have to teach ourselves, through loosening up exercises and positive attitudes – not by any artificial attempt to force it – to let our poise return.

(ix) The Head should Balance Lightly, and Lead the Spine Up

Ever since the earliest single cell animals began to acquire a front and a rear end, the head has led animal movement; and the human head still needs to be aware of its leading *up-front* or now *up-top* position. Our own head needs a light balance and a very slight forwardness as it leads the spine in its upward lengthening. It is a good idea to forget about head position, for it is not a fixed but a dynamic, upward-directed balance.

If you are familiar with the Alexander Technique, you will know about this lightness and its importance to the whole body. A skilled Alexander teacher can guide this upward lengthening lightly with his or her hands. But even unaided we can become increasingly aware, as F.M. Alexander did himself, of our length and balance. We can give ourselves reminders and consciously *lighten up*. Ask yourself sometimes: "Is my head compressing my neck?", and then ask it to stop doing that.

The Zen teacher Shunryu Suzuki says that when the chin is tilted up we are probably dreaming. Posture, sitting or standing or in movement is very important to Zen and other Buddhists. They intuitively value its *rightness*. This is not mentioned in Zen and the Art of Motorcycling, but posture must be important to motorcyclists as well. I have seen and admired some beautiful pillion riding sometimes.

Somehow we seem to be only fully present to the here and now when the balance of the head is light and free. For the head to balance freely, the neck vertebrae should never be locked. The neck is not a separate limb and we need to be free to use it always as part of the longer spine.

But there is another aspect of necks that should also influence the amount of respect we give them and that is the neck's development as a channel and container, not just as a sort of plinth to stand the head on. The voice box lives in the throat and it works better when it has plenty of space and is not squashed. So do all the blood vessels and tubes and nerves that carry nutrients and oxygen and messages, down into the body and especially up into the brain. When we give better operating conditions to these supply lines, we make better use of our brain and all the essential sensing apparatus housed in the head. This dual role of containing and channelling obviously works best when the head is very lightly balanced.

It is important to look after all the delicate apparatus of the senses. All our information from the world around us comes to us through this amazing equipment, and it is essential to be well informed about our surroundings. If we think about it we recognise that fine sensing – and this applies to hands too – depends upon free and sensitive mobility. All the supply lines of nerves and blood vessels need to be open and the sensory equipment in the head needs to be sensitively supported and balanced and free to move easily. The quality of our experience of the whole of life is affected by this fine balance of the head on the spinal column.

Our ability to make any contact at all with our environment seems miraculous. Little by little we have been able to interpret it, use it and even appreciate, husband and care for it. This faculty evolved in movement. We must have bumped into millions of obstacles before acquiring these incredibly sensitive ways of sorting out our surroundings. Starting with the intimate close-up senses of taste and touch, powered by some basic chemistry and physics, the earliest organisms began to develop a much bigger range of senses. They found ways to extract more and more information from further and further away. We now use information carried by airborne molecules and the pressure of sound waves and the photons of light across larger and larger distances, in the faculties of scent, sound and sight.

We taste best when the tongue moves around. We interpret and communicate best with touch when we can explore sensitively with touching. We smell, hear and see best when our head is free to move very slightly around the molecules or the sound and light waves we are using. A free neck makes all of this sensing truly sensitive. It allows us to experience a much deeper pleasure from the scent of a rose garden, or from music or landscape, or anything else, than we could possibly receive from a clamped head position. There is a richer experience in exploring around any signals that come our way.

We even communicate verbally more openly and fully with other people when the head is not fixed. Our voice and eyes can roam a little in their direction. It is not socially helpful to face the other person with a fixed and glassy stare like that of the Ancient Mariner because they sense and react to such rigidity. Singers instinctively use facial and body movement. If they stand stiffly we feel much less moved by their performance. Visual staring seems to cut us off. *Vocal staring,* too, the "undirected monologue of the bore" as Patsy Rodenburg describes the voice that drones on and on, also cuts us off from the sensitive experience of being with the other person. A similar whole body withdrawal can happen subconsciously and diminish our entire reception of information from our environment. We then miss useful feed-back, as well as all the sensory pleasure we could be having from the world around us.

So the carriage of the head is important. If we think of the neck as needing to be three dimensionally open and free, to care for its contents, as well as flexible and light for fluid movement, and upright for self esteem and openness to others, and for carrying the sense organs and voice efficiently, we can become increasingly considerate about the way we hold that balance.

Maybe this elaboration of the value of a lightly balanced head has been rather lengthy, but awareness begins with such searching and thinking, and exploring what may be involved. It then starts a process that gradually allows us to let go of our minor thrusts, tilts and tensions one by one. You can use these pictures as awareness triggers to free up your neck at odd moments, even if you never take exercise!

Because anxiety about one's head position is counter productive, my chosen neck exercises are loose and pleasurable and almost lazily relaxed.

(x) Natural Movement Flows

When any animal is reaching out or leaping, exploring or searching, movement flows right through the body. This is so for millipedes, quadrupeds, starfish, jellyfish, spiders, cats and horses and all forms of life. Even bipeds share out their movements around the muscles of the two sides, and snakes send ripples all the way from head to tail. We, too, are naturally supple and should aim to be flexible in every joint and muscle to make this grace and fluidity possible.

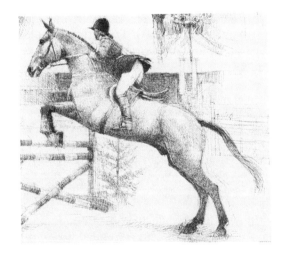

Extension from top to toe (William Geldart)

This elegance is nature's way of sharing mechanical effort around the body's structure as a whole. It creates minimum strain and gives maximum ease and efficiency. Like poised stillness, graceful movement is a pleasing bonus of efficiency.

There is something especially pleasing in the flow of human creative and expressive movement in the use of tools, a specifically human development. We sense something that we can call *spirit* in action, as if that fluent movement communicates across the gap between people. A pancake maker in any kitchen, or a skilled craftsman at work with an adze, loom or potter's wheel, communicates a joy in those creative activities that reaches out to others. We respond with pleasure.

Actors know well that bodily movement in any action, somehow carries a person's unique individual creative expressiveness, and audiences respond to this directly. We are drawn to natural grace and are repelled by the awkwardness that is there when this flow is absent. Even musical expressiveness in singing and playing as well as conducting is rooted in the body.

When aware of this quality of individual personal expressiveness and the way it communicates, we can encourage the flow of our own movement, right through the main frame of the body and out of the fingertips or the voice, or through a brush, pen, chisel or instrument, wherever we are expressing or enjoying ourselves, whether as craftsmen, singers, actors or musicians, or just taking a walk or talking with friends. Not with excessive flourish perhaps, unless we are opera singers or dramatic actors, but aware that even a modest fluidity lets us tune in to ourselves and to reach across to the other person.

This ability to cross boundaries is a spiritual aspect of flow. It bridges the gap between us. The inner urge to communicate, whether our happiness or sadness, our love, lust or fury, uses the natural flow of released and supple muscles.

At the receiving end too, we need a non-tense receptivity or *listening*. Just as a stiff, inhibited or untrained skill does not come across to us as powerfully as one that flowed confidently from the voice, brush, tool or instrument of its creator, so also our own enjoyment of an art or craft is enhanced when our body is relaxed and sensitively mobile. The difference is one of quality, like that between death and life.

(xi) The Three Dimensions Extend Together

Length and width have been discussed separately, but we really need to extend into the 3-Dness of every scrap of our body. Alive animals are *Expanding Universes*, not *White Dwarf Stars*. The whole body's length, depth and width is being continuously maintained, all the time we live, all of it together, in this extension.

Living life to the full seems to require a lightly expanding outward pressure, right to the three-dimensional detail of every cell and every joint, and, for good measure, some multi-dimensional extension for the mind and human spirit, too. Perhaps this necessary outward physical pressure of adventurous life · accounts for the importance we give to the positive in all the other spheres of our actions, speech-actions and attitudes. Extension is part of life itself – a primary plus.

If you think about it, you can feel this sense of positive expansion in your own body while reading these words. We are able to give our bodies this awareness of the 3-D space they inhabit. In a later visualisation exercise we can explore this in some detail.

Breathing fully is one important and observable part of our creation of our full quota of space; positive attitudes, happiness, a positive outlook and a happy and exuberant spirit are others. Imagine you are greeting an old friend, really happy to see her, and you open up your arms, your face, and the whole body for a greeting and embrace. You probably take in a huge breath while you do that, and then radiate your pleasure in expansive body and words. "How wonderful to see you!" Such natural happiness, extending outwards and sparkling, is a real tonic for bodies, minds and spirits.

3-D shrinkage is the harmful opposite of this condition and we need to correct for it consciously. If you really must clench a fist in anger, do shake it loose afterwards. Massage your hands, wrists, neck and face sometimes too, to bring them back to their unstressed natural condition.

Affectionate touching extends us. It softens and releases muscles. When we kiss a child's hurt knee, or smooth it gently to make it better, we help both the child and ourselves to some physical and psychological release. She is helped to let go of the surge of physical tension that came as she shrank from the hurt. Her own healing powers become freed again as she opens up and feels comforted. We expand a little as well, from having helped her. The pain goes away and she is not left with tightened muscles or a lasting fear. The emotional release exercise of a later chapter can help us even now to let go of such ancient fears of our own when we have not been helped at the time.

(xii) The Quadruped Factor

Human bodies have inherited traces of many interesting earlier muscular systems. We can still squirm and wriggle if we want to, or writhe in pain if we need to, just like our invertebrate ancestors. But one major pattern of movement is still very important to us and that is the quite recent quadrupedal arrangement that coordinates the use of the right forelimb with that of the left hind limb and vice versa.

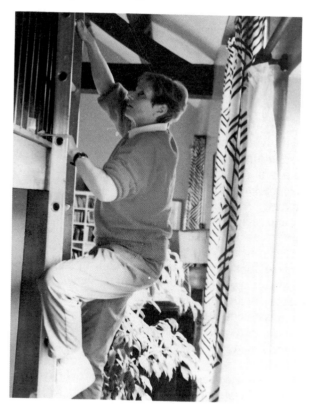

Climbing uses the four limbs quadrupedally.
(The author taking an alternative route upstairs.)

We have linked muscles that spiral round the body maintaining this quadrupedal connection. We are bipedal quadrupeds, or quadrupeds with some recent advantageous adaptations, not an original and symmetrically two-sided design.

Although the human two-legged animal can use all four limbs in different ways, as in driving a car, for example, yet we can still feel the links between a shoulder and the opposite hip as we walk or climb or swim. The division across the human brain plays a part in this ancient organisation of body movements, since each hemisphere is managing movement on the opposite side of the body. So whenever our limbs are using their criss-cross connections, we necessarily involve both sides of the brain at once. In deliberate coordination exercises we can gently force a cooperation between them as if prising open some rusty brain connections.

Because we no longer walk quadrupedally, the left and right brains may come to believe they don't need each other, and to some extent this is so. Modern human bodies are comparatively well protected and secure in most civilised communities and we can get away with a measure of clumsiness. Our life no longer depends on high levels of bodily skill and we don't need good coordination to survive.

Yet, as we have seen, a mental dominance of either the left or right is not desirable in the brain's management. So mentally as well as physically it is valuable to exercise to minimise our own clumsiness across the body and at the same time work to strengthen this basic coordination within our nervous system. Watch a cat stalking its prey and you see this alertness and very deliberate four-footedness in action together, all of its energy and purpose heading towards one focused aim.

(xiii) Breathing: Our Interface with the Universe

It is impossible to arrange this catalogue of evolved expectations in any right order. Perhaps breathing should have come first. Fresh air is vital to us. We can imagine that we have a living contract with our universe/environment in the business of breath. I see my lungs almost as a placenta in this relationship between me and my universe. All the time, we have a full exchange of ingredients going on, from and back into the air around us. The rest of the body then draws upon and organises its use of the life giving oxygen.

The thorax is not a rigid cage but an elastic and welcoming structure making the best use of this primary relationship between the organism and its environment. If we breathe minimally we deprive ourselves of the generous supply of oxygen and vitality that our universe is offering. But when we breathe fully and naturally we optimise this essential flow to body and brain. It is good to remind ourselves of this basic interdependence from time to time, even of our actual oneness with our environment while we live and breathe, and our many responsibilities towards it.

The breathing exercises I have chosen use gentle movements of body weight and limbs. Large movements, even quite gentle ones, extend the body's demand for oxygen and bring a natural expansion of the rib cage in natural movement. We should not bring a forced, exaggerated muscular activity to breathing.

(xiv) We also Need to Rest

Like breathing, rest is so obviously important to bodies that it seems wrong to speak of it last. We are programmed to expect rest and to benefit from it. But it needs few words, perhaps just a nod of recognition here, and a recommendation to include relaxation in any fitness campaign.

We are capable of periods of extreme exertion and need the balance of deeply satisfying rest between these. A good programme of regular exercise makes us more fit to make demands on our bodies, but we must respect this complementary basic need of all animal life if we are to be wholly fit, and find our own best way to enjoy times of relaxation and recuperation.

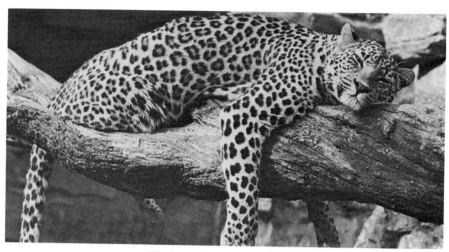

We also need to rest (Chester Zoo)

Saying 'Yes' to Evolution

Even without any deliberate periods of exercise, our physical and mental health improve just from awareness and acknowledgement of these fourteen basic evolutionary expectations that our biological history brings with it. We know then what our body expects of us and can agree to supply it with all these. But we can reinforce that awareness with exercises. They bring us into the here and now and remind us of our body's pleasures and possibilities as well as its basic needs.

Neglect never kills us outright, but little by little prolonged neglect or mistakenly damaging exercise will cut back on the quality of our life as a whole. When we build on the most positive basics we can use all the liveliest parts of that inheritance in the best ways. Our life style is affected by the whole of our history, genetic and personal, of course, and also by whatever immediate activity we are engaged in right at this very moment. There may be some quite small improvement we could be offering as a gift to show our appreciation of this inheritance.

Don't imagine these principles are restrictive. They bring us great freedom. The best freedom always needs rules in the same way that a kite needs its string. It is quite easy to incorporate a cheerful recognition of them all into our everyday lives. You can get value from them just by re-reading this guideline list, even just the headings, from time to time and saying a firm "Yes!" as you make each one very fully your own.

Become your own expert in putting these principles to good use. Simple and obvious as they are, they should be a practical guide to all of us at all times.

Principles and practice are useless apart. They have a Jacob's Ladder relationship. There is movement up and down between them all the time. What we do about them is just as important as the principles and that is where exercise comes in.

Fortunately, Evolution Does Not Limit the Spirit!

The human spirit has to express itself through the body and mind, and to that extent it does have some earthbound limitations! But as spirit is an abstract term it is not a product of our genes and so need not be limited much by the processes of our evolution. It can create its forward visions and direct its positive energies purposefully towards strengthening its best of human qualities wherever and in whatever circumstances it finds itself. Evolution could not act in a teleological way. People can. The future is quite different in quality from the past and we can act to make it brighter.

As spirits have no DNA, no genetic instructions and no mechanical problems at all, we can always be imaginatively creative about exercising this part of our team. The exercises I suggest in a later chapter are not meant to be limitations but launching pads for spirits. You can go as high and as far as you choose once you accept a spiritual dimension.

If the body/mind entity were spiritless, then, left to its own devices, groping about, looking for niches to exploit, and unaware of any *top-down* possibilities, it could easily operate entirely selfishly. It could assume that ancient and primitive strategies for trampling over others for personal gain are the best practices for human beings! Many modern feuding societies and criminals everywhere are still doing this and so are many of us in one way and another, just as some earlier primate societies did. But when we give some body/mind house room to the human spirit, aware human beings balance self caring with a bigger involvement with other people and all of life. We are able to use abstract and spiritual ideas to make this switch away from complete self-centredness.

As spirits have no need to look towards the past at all, except where it inspires, teaches or perhaps entertains them, when it comes to exercising our spirits, we can reverse Darwinism with a flourish. Goodbye evolution! Goodbye chance! Hello responsible, positive and creative forward action!

The past will always, in any case, look as though it was totally produced by chance, however dazzling its pageant and results, and that can feel dispiriting. The future is an entirely different commodity! We can be creatively constructive about it. Exercise expands our opportunities for doing that.

3

Guidelines from The Mechanics: The "Owner's Manual" Approach

All the evolutionary guidelines are vital ones, but there are other pointers to good bodily usage. Human lives have changed so much that today we also need some up-to-date guidance from the newer left brain skills. Both logic and mechanical understanding can help us. Without being experts we can learn a great deal from our knowledge of simple engineering principles.

If we were machines, though we know we are much more than that, how could we minimise the wear of these machines and maximise the duration of their health and life, as responsible body owners? We may be complete amateurs in our knowledge of evolution or of engineering, but we can profit from using even the simplest pictures from these two approaches.

(i) Oil the Joints and Hinges

An obvious first when we use any machinery, bicycle, car or sewing machine, is that all the places of articulation should be lubricated. What does this mean for our personal body machine?

In the world of nature, joints are *oiled* in the plentiful everyday movements of hunting for foods, building nests and so on. The natural joint lubricant that does this job, the synovial fluid, also brings vital oxygen to the living cells of the joints. Today's humans often limit their daily movement enormously, and a habit of regular under-use leads both to drying of joints and to oxygen starvation. Driving to the supermarket and pushing a trolley are not really enough! Perhaps we should install warning lights to let us know when more lubrication, that is, more easy unstressed moving around, is needed!

Excess tension, when moving or stationary, even if quite slight, damages joints because it narrows the access for these lubricants. Loosening up exercises and deliberate pauses for deep relaxation as well as plentiful light movement, all help to release these restrictions so that the natural *oiling* can go on. Local tightness in machine or man also has more general effects on the structure as a whole. Slowly and surely the ability of the mechanism to react quickly is damped. We have the same loss of mechanical efficiency when we drive a car with the brakes on, or a bicycle with no oil in the bearings. The exercises of this programme take you through easy but important loosening/lubricating movements for just about every joint in the body.

(ii) Stack the Main Weights Wisely

A mechanical structure of any height will obviously balance best when its main masses are stacked vertically one above the other. As quite young children soon learn with their building blocks, a vertical axis is practical. For the human biped, we can think of the stationary balance either as piled up – see Figure A1 in the Alignment Diagram of Chapter 4 – or suspended from the sky – as in Figure A3. If we introduce a lean we introduce a strain and need to return to that sensible alignment again.

These two mechanical images of uprightness work together. We are, at the same time, both firmly grounded on earth by the gravitational forces, and, oppositely, with our anti-gravity muscles working, we are lightly extended upwards out of it. Oriental traditions have used such an image for thousands of years and still value its metaphorical extras. Being rooted on a very solid planet reminds us of our animal origins, and being also directed upwards we remember the higher spiritual values of our culture.

We can use this image of a double directedness to throw light on many other dualities in our lives. We are juggling with opposites all the time and this image gives us a broad perspective on many of our very interesting challenges.

(iii) Avoid Rigidity

As well as *oiling* the joints with easy movement, we need to maintain the health and general resilience of the whole body machine. The muscular system is involved as well as the joints. We are designed to move and to do so smoothly and lightly, and it is the muscles which do this work by contracting and releasing. Our joints are virtually friction-free when we are moving well. But stiff muscles, like unlubricated joints, hamper all the natural processes of walking running and jumping.

We need to give our muscles frequent opportunities to work over their full range and we should stretch them gently when they have been under or overused to keep this range available. Well exercised muscles will then always be available to move the joints easily at any time and give the skeletal structure its fullest support. It is interesting how noticeable other people's stiffnesses are, as well as our own. We immediately notice the unnaturalness of it. In nature, stiff or awkward movement would indicate vulnerability, and the life of the stiff person would be at risk to sharp eyed predators.

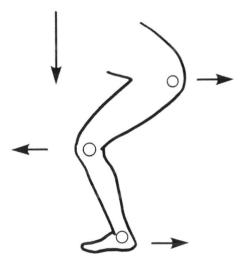

The hinges at ankle, knee and hip that lower the whole body vertically

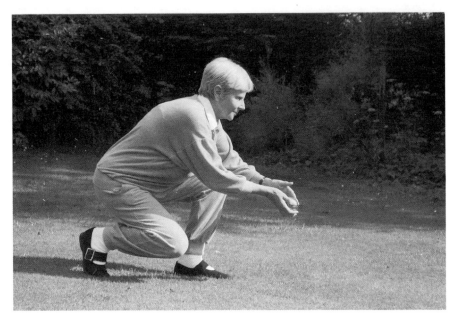

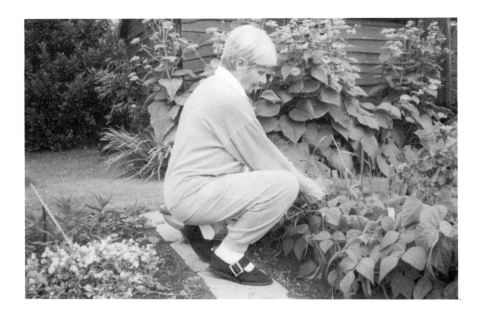

For playing boules or picking beans, the hinges at hip, knee and ankle save the back from strain.
Flexible feet increase the possibilities

(iv) Make Use of the Hinges

Legs effectively have three strong mechanical hinges, in the ankles knees and hip joints. There is also a hinge of sorts across the line of the toe joints, one that we use for walking and running and from which we can lift to stand on our toes. These are perfect for raising and lowering the rest of the body and they work together as we move around in the world's three dimensions. It is important to keep all these hinges well exercised, the joints regularly loosened over a full range of movement, and the muscles that operate them released and well toned. If we under-use and so grow stiff in our ankles and knees, or if we over-tighten leg muscles and buttocks, we may jam up the hip joint and spoil the natural springiness of walking.

The nearest approach to a hinge in the spine is in the small top vertebra on which the skull pivots, and there is no other. Apart from this local high up pivot called the atlas, and the extra rotation available in the axis vertebra below it, for larger movements the whole of the neck should operate in one with the spine. To lower the head simply vertically we can use ankle, knee and hip hinges, and let the whole upright back descend. Or to curve downwards, forwards or back, we start at the tiny top rocking hinge and then gradually use more of the spine's flexibility to extend further. For a rotation, the turning also starts very high and then brings in the rest of the spine as required. It can continue all the way down, around a vertical axis, like a spiral staircase, using waist, hips, knees and ankles, too, if we need to look right behind us.

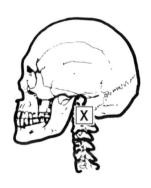

The pivot for the head is high up at the very top of the spine, marked with "X".

There is no hinge in the middle of either the neck or the back. We have quite a lot of flexibility in the human spine and it is valuable to look after this with exercises, but we get into mechanical trouble in these two places if we habitually hold a forward or backward lean or bend or thrust at the waist or upper back or neck. These result in a break in the alignment and an awkwardly tense carriage of the main weights of the body.

A primary engineering safeguard for every body's back, is to keep the three leg hinges free and strong with exercise, and then use them more deliberately as we lower the whole body to reach into low cupboards or pick things up from the floor. We can find out in aware exercising exactly where the leg hinges are. We can get to know where the top atlas vertebra is too, and we can learn to notice our use of these joints and protect the spine by using them all well.

(v) Don't Skew the Arches

Arches are strong engineering structures. The mechanical principle of the arch as a strong supporting and load-spreading device, was a great discovery of the early Roman engineers, but nature discovered it first. Many invertebrate animals can arch their bodies and the human skeleton has several bony arches. The human body machine is a living and moving structure so there is some flexibility available at the main structural places of our arches and the body as a whole can move efficiently and adjust its balance safely over them.

I have stressed the value of recognising some asymmetry in the evolved human form, but here in its arch structures, the sheer mechanics does impose a need for at least a partially localised symmetry. We must use their flexibility that is available whenever we need it, but we should not let an habitual skewing or leaning put a permanent distorting torque or bending pressure on to any of our arches.

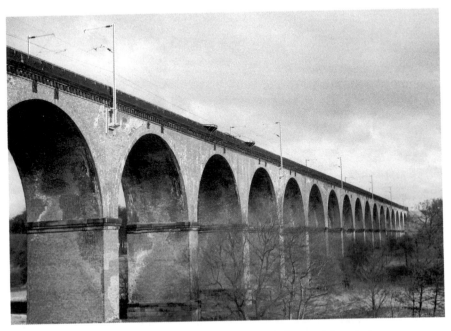

Arches are very strong structures: the vertical alignment is important

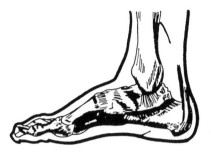

THE LONGITUDINAL ARCH

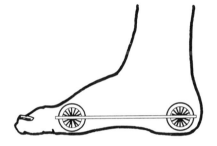

AS IF ON FOUR WHEELS

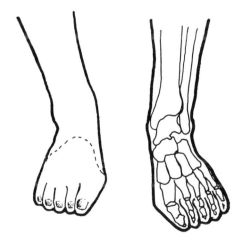

THE TRANSVERSE ARCH FORMED
FROM BONES LINKED ACROSS
THE FOOT

SPREADING THE LOAD

The arches of the feet give a strong flexible resilient base for the whole of the body's weight. Each foot is arched in length and also in width and we should carry our weight down the leg bones over the strongest part of this vaulting. A good approximation is to load the foot fairly centrally, as if on four roller skate wheels, all evenly loaded. When we habitually stand or walk with skewed feet or ankles, the local unbalance goes all the way up. Wearing shoes is an unavoidable restriction for modern feet and we need to work regularly on the flexibility of arches as well as ankles to compensate for this necessary everyday restriction.

The human body also uses its two legs and the pelvis bridging them, rather

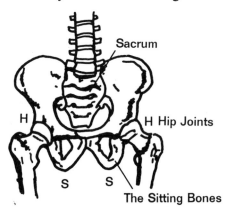

like a tall, quite narrow arch, above and at right angles to the main arches of the feet. The hip joints are only a few inches apart, set deeply into the pelvis. They are not at the bony extremity that we often think of as the hip joint, nor higher in the pelvis which sometimes gets confusingly labelled as the hip bone.

The pelvis as arch: weight is carried between the hip joints (H) when standing. When sitting, there is effectively an arch above the sitting bones, S.

When aware of this tall main supporting structure as a narrow arch, we can see the sense of finding a comfortably balanced, non-leaning, resting stance, and a walking posture with the feet not in line, but just a little way apart.

The sacrum acts as the keystone of this pelvic arch. We need to stay quite flexible, but not kinked, at the important structural point where spine and sacrum meet because of the continuous balancing process in which we are involved. If the legs are uneven in length, or just for a comfortable standing position, a slightly wider stance may give a more restful balance. Think of carrying the weight of the upper body through the spine which rises vertically above the vertical arch of the pelvis.

When we sit, a different pelvic arch supports the spine. This time, two bony knobs at the bottom of the pelvis, the ischial tuberosities, or sitting bones, form the base of the arch, and the sacrum is again its keystone. The sitting bones are closer to the mid-line than the hip joints are, so this is an even narrower arch.

Again, above this sitting base, the pelvis should not angle forwards or tuck hard under, but balance uprightly, especially if we are at work at a desk or table. Our legs and feet are also usually on the ground when we sit, and they take part in the balancing act. It is best to sit evenly, usually with the legs uncrossed and a little apart, the feet feeling the ground and the buttocks free of tension. Think of *standing* on the sitting bones, balancing head above broad shoulders above vertical pelvis.

The costal or ribcage arch is not structural in the same way as the arch of legs and pelvis and is not joined to that arch directly, but stands above it, supported by the spine, rather like a proud second tier in a Roman viaduct. If we habitually lean or twist this arch of the ribs we may develop some rigidity in the rib cage and can strain the upper spine and also the hip and lumbar joints.

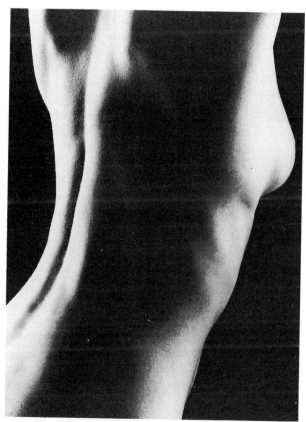

When walking we should not sink the ribs closer to the pelvis as we step, but let the upward thrust of our walk and the fullness of breathing help to keep this arch naturally high above the pelvis.

(vi) Keep The Midriff Elastic, Long and Strong

The abdominal muscles play an important role in the body's overall mechanics. Firstly, they are needed to contain all the food processing equipment, and for women, the space for a baby to grow in, so both strength and elasticity are necessary.

They are also needed for holding the

Length, strength and suppleness are the vital ingredients for mid-section fitness *(Michael Busselle)* weight of those contents towards the spine for greatest mechanical efficiency. Weight carried too far out from the structural main axis puts a great strain on the muscles and ligaments that have to carry it.

The abdominals also play a less direct part in supporting the spine. If we collapse our length here, they pull down in such a way that the spine has a hard time maintaining its proper length and flexibility. The spinal vertebrae then, including those of the neck, may wear excessively and eventually painfully.

When anything has to be expelled from the body, such as a foreign body from the throat or lungs, or when vomiting is necessary, or emptying the bladder or bowel, these muscles may be involved. Our breath and our voice are powered here, too, and suffer noticeably if we let this section collapse.

There are three main sets of abdominal muscles, the longitudinal, transverse and oblique ones together forming an elastic cylinder. This strong sheath of multi-layered muscles stays long and quite well toned if we are plentifully active, running, jumping and climbing. We know that sitting for a long time, and especially sitting badly, compresses and harms this abdominal corset, but we may damage it even more when we strengthen it in compression, as in some hunched sit-up exercises. Unless we have extremely fit abdominals, exercises that

RIBS

PELVIS

PUBIC BONE

(i)   THE ABDOMINAL 'CORSET' ATTACHES TO RIBS, PELVIC RIM AND PUBIC BONE.

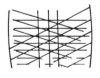

(ii)   PROPORTIONS ARE EXAGGERATED HERE TO SHOW HOW COLLAPSED ABDOMINALS SHORTEN AND WIDEN THIS SECTION. THE SPINE LOSES RESILIENCE. BREATHING SUFFERS. APPEARANCE TOO IS NOT ENHANCED.

train them for strength while they are shortened, will tend to bring the rib cage closer to the pelvis and so compress the spine and squash the inner organs.

If we lead a very sedentary life, bursts of sit-ups are not the best way to help these muscles. We need awareness of the job they are doing, active use of them in much of our everyday movement and regular sound exercises specifically to tone them gently.

(vii) Respect the Asymmetry

The human body machine is not driven by clockwork and does not have exact bilateral symmetry. If we had evolved differently, as bipeds from the very start of life, with left and right sides exactly matching and muscles and nerves running up and down the two sides completely symmetrically, we would never adopt any distorting bodily twists. Instead, as we have seen, we have muscle linkages in our structure that form continuous spirals around the body.

Internally, heart and stomach, liver and lungs are all arranged unsymmetrically. Some of us may also have one leg shorter than the other, or have adopted a slight twist from a particular sport or a childhood habit. Or we may have had accidents to one limb or one side of the body, adding even more unevennesses to our normal slight asymmetry.

We have wonderful bi-pedal freedom available, but it is not good mechanics to force a rigid symmetry on this structure, either in our exercises or in everyday usage. Forcing and jarring, especially with repetitive movement, increase tensions and can perpetuate a fault that began as a temporary or quite minor imbalance. Twisting the body while working it quite hard is another hazard for us. It is always a good safeguard to turn the feet and legs and all our attention in the direction of any strong arm movement we want to make, such as opening a heavy door or even flushing a toilet cistern.

Managing this interesting asymmetry and all its possibilities involves staying aware of the hazards of misuse. We can learn a lot from watching animal movement and see how the big apes or other nearly bi-pedal animals use their bodies really freely but never foolishly. We can also help by using almost continuous very slight movement, even while sitting or standing, and talking or listening, to keep this non-symmetrical structure unlocked all over.

When model girls are taught to walk very symmetrically, bringing the feet to a central line, they inevitably introduce pelvic stresses which very high heeled shoes then aggravate. The natural alignment of hip, leg and foot lies just outside the body's mid-line and we have to force it a little, possibly straining the hip joints if we try to bring every step round to the centre.

Each leg in turn has to support the whole body and the weight of the heavy head, and we need a slight transfer from side to side and a slight up and down movement as we walk. We can see this sometimes in slow motion film of a crowd walking rhythmically. There is a 3-D aspect to our walk that enlivens its general linearity. The faster the walk the closer our feet will come to a central line. And with an average, fairly lively pace, each forward thrust provides enough momentum for us to stay almost airborne between the moments of touchdown.

Tucking the pelvis in tightly is another locking action that distorts a natural leg swing and can damage hip and back joints. If modelling clothes brings you these occupational risks, do loosen up regularly with a lot of much freer movements. Climb a few trees!

Our bi-pedalism has freed us to walk in very many ways, including frog-walking, Cossack dancing, goose-stepping and other military variations, but the human machine should avoid any prolonged exercise that feels like clockwork. Clocks have brought enough restrictions to human bodily freedom, without us imitating their precision in stylised walking. Find some tussocks or rocks and boulders to negotiate on walks, and choose rough hill walking as a change from concrete pavements and crowded shopping malls.

Our walk, like our posture, is very personally and distinctively our own. It can be beautifully poised and free if we respect the needs of the mechanics of the structure and give it the variety it enjoys.

(viii) Maintain the Pumps and Circulation Systems

The two obvious mechanical pumps of the body machine are the heart and the lungs which keep beating and breathing, non-stop, for as long as we live. And the main requirements for these are mostly a sufficiently free space to work in, open supply lines, non rigid ribs, sound nutrition and plenty of exercise. With good conditions they will operate powerfully for a long lifetime.

But the muscles of our limbs also act to some extent as pumps. These big muscles assist actively with the circulation of the blood in all the movements they make. This includes locomotion, for legs, and all the work we do with our arms. They are, therefore, also involved in transporting oxygen and vital nutrients to cells, muscles and brain, and in removing waste products from these. When muscles are under-used these processes are damaged by the stagnation that follows. Animal hearts did not evolve in a stationary machine, doing all the work alone like a beam engine. They were always part of a system in almost continual extension and overall movement in which every muscle worked with regular cycles of contraction and release.

The lymph system is also *pumped* in its own way, removing waste via the sweat glands and skin. This needs plenty of fresh water to keep the processes of diffusion active around every cell and it, too, needs movement to assist these processes. Spinal fluids as well are circulated only by our movements and stagnate if the spine just sits about. We need to get up and walk and carry our own weight around for the sake of everything that circulates and flows in us.

Climbing and swimming are excellent ways of maintaining all the pumping systems of the body, using the large muscles of all four limbs together, and flexing and twisting the spine in healthy movement. Walking and running use mostly the pumping action of the leg muscles, but as these are the biggest muscles their contribution is very important and these are excellent exercises for the cardiovascular system.

Armchairs, on the other hand, may be more dangerous than we think, especially if we become addicted to them. Prolonged sitting reduces the circulation to a gentle tick-over which, though natural at night and for reasonable periods of rest, cannot possibly maintain our optimum circulatory fitness on its own, long-term. After half an hour of sitting, any self respecting body machine needs to walk about, run somewhere, do some stretches or gardening or climb some stairs to keep these pumps and the whole circulation system in good condition.

If we think about the mechanical needs of our body's pumping systems we will want to provide them with a balance of natural rest and healthy considerate exercise, sufficient oxygen, fresh water and wholesome food as fuel. They will certainly respond well to our intelligent caring in these matters. If we think about exercise as a kind of nutrition for bodies we can teach ourselves to supply these fundamental needs sensibly.

(ix) What About Fuel?

The evolutionary pointers to good fuel would be to use fresh fruits and vegetables and grains as a large part of our diet since they have served the species well for millions of years. Plants have evolved ways to carry all the minerals we need from the soil, and we have evolved an ability to use their carbohydrate and mineral contents to construct and power our bodies. We can also use the more concentrated protein foods from animal meat, but this should play a smaller part than the simpler plant foods.

If we look at fuel needs simply from the aspect of providing good mechanical conditions for the body, there are also common sense guidelines here for our choices.

Some foods have the property of *sludging* the blood, and thus cutting down its oxygen-carrying capacity. Excesses of animal fats do this. Then, however efficient and well exercised the pumps, circulation will gradually be hampered from within and the heart and brain and all other organs will be poorly supplied.

It also makes sense to maximise the ways in which we can give our whole body the oxygen it vitally needs. Sensible mechanical guidelines include breathing fully, of course, especially outside in the fresh air, avoiding smoking or smoky environments, avoiding toxic or fatty clogging foods, and keeping plenty of everyday movement for both the skeleton and the digestive processes. These practical steps and some well chosen exercises will ensure the oxygen supply necessary to keep muscles and joints, the immune system and all mental functioning in good shape.

The human species has flourished because it is so amazingly adaptable. It can obviously survive moderate levels of nutritional abuse, just as a machine can be made to work with low grade fuel. But it makes much better sense to provide our bodies with the best possible natural foods and the purest water. A perfectionist would watch every detail of nutritional intake and eschew everything containing chemically harmful additives. But even a moderate vigilance is better than none. Any nutritional change in a positive direction, however small, is well worth making.

The other simple but very practical mechanical factor relating to fuel supplies is not to overload the digestive system with excessive bulk of foods, however good! Some of us need this information more than others, but it is true that, as Anna Russell said: "If it is too much it is too much, even if it is ni-i-i-ce!"

Eating quite lightly is one of the best contributions we can make to the body's mechanical efficiency. A heavily overloaded gut puts a big local strain on the spine, and unless our energy output is very big, we have the longer term mechanical hazard of storing too much fat and acquiring an excessive accumulation of weight to carry around. So many psychological and emotional factors can affect our desire for food that good guidelines and the intervention of consciousness are increasingly necessary to influence our choices.

(x) The Sensitive Machine

A well-tuned engine is so much more responsive than a rusty one, that there are clear rewards in doing anything we can to improve our body's mechanical efficiency. The more finely tuned it is, the more closely it will be in touch with its real needs, and will let us know of them. Starting out from a basic respect for the body's alignment, and a few common sense engineering basics, we quite simply become more sensitive in a holistic way.

Extending the metaphor a little, as our antennae become more sensitive, we increasingly tune in more accurately to the needs of others as well as ourselves, and even to the needs of the important environment that supports and nourishes us. If you do not think that sensitivity could ever come from such practical issues as mechanical soundness, just put these ordinary mechanical principles into your life, act on them and see what happens!

Choose the Best: Choose the Plus and Stay Awake!

Maybe the biggest choice for fitness, even at the mechanical level, is the positive one of wanting to have the *machine* working all the time at its best possible level. This is infinitely better than looking only at the negative aspect of rescuing it from time to time, like an old banger, from collapse and corrosion, or trying to train it for fighting or for competition it will never have to face. This positive goal represents a totally different approach. Don't wait for the problem that often brings people to exercise classes. How much more positive and realistic to work towards better than average functioning and switch some of your awareness to your day-to-day and DIY maintenance. You may not become problem free, but problems will be more rare, as in a well maintained car.

Every slight shift of mental attitude towards a more actively positive care of one's body machine brings big dividends. Sitting in a better chair when the one you are using forces you to slump, opening up the body instead of closing it down; or sometimes choosing an apple instead of cake, or water instead of whisky, does make a positive difference to our well-being, and to the work we do.

It should be a part of our everyday common sense to give this Rolls Royce of a body the very best chance to serve us well. We know very well that we are not just machines, and yet in one basic sense this piece of mechanics is all that we have! It deserves respect and regular care. Become your own expert. Use these practical guidelines to wake up to a new appreciation of the very fine instrument or vehicle you have. After all, you are not just looking after yourself. Everything we do for this *machine* makes possible a bigger contribution to other people and to all that we value in life.

4

Postural Alignment and Proprioception

The Head, Body and Legs Diagrams

The three main blocks of the body's weight balance best simply one above the other – see Figures A1 and A2. If this seems obvious, look around and see how often that line is distorted.

In any deflection from this alignment we have to use extra effort to manage the extra strains and pressures that the forces of gravity bring to bear.

We can also help our anti-gravity system of muscles by imagining we are suspended from the sky above, our length extended, with all the weight bearing joints open and free rather than compressed down (Figure A3). We can also help by imagining our whole spine lengthening upwards, shoulders out to the sides and resting downwards, and the crown of the head extending towards the sky.

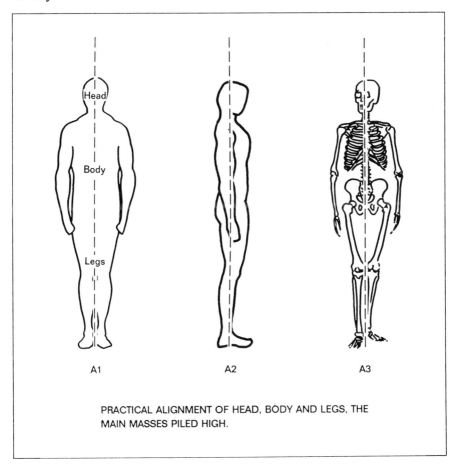

A1   A2   A3

PRACTICAL ALIGNMENT OF HEAD, BODY AND LEGS, THE
MAIN MASSES PILED HIGH.

Weight each foot fairly evenly as if on four non-skewed roller skate wheels. Allow them both to spread and lengthen and to feel the floor. Balance the head lightly. Don't lock the knees. The ischial bones at the bottom of the pelvis are directed to the floor, neither tucked hard under nor pushed hard back. Our stationary balance is most efficient when these building blocks are vertically aligned like this, head above body above legs. And the most efficient way of turning round is also to rotate around the vertical axis right through these, rather than bending as we turn.

Making Friends with Gravity – Some Alignment Considerations

The vertical lines of Figures B1, 2, 3 and 4 represent the lines of the force of gravity. These are our best guide to finding a good neutral line to return to. Imagine them raining down around you. When standing, if the main weights of head, body and legs are nicely lined up and balanced one above the other, all that weight is carried efficiently by the whole foot. It descends through the bones and is carried lightly above the arches made from the heel and the spread of the bones of the rest of the foot. Feet have a lot of sensors and we can become more and more aware of the way they are carrying our weight.

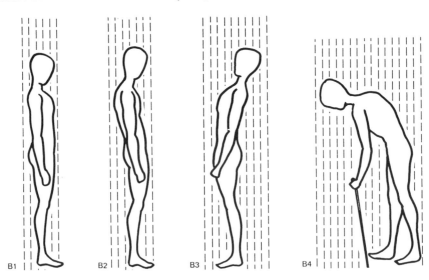

TENSION IS INTRODUCED WHENEVER WE LEAVE THE BALANCED ALIGNMENT. EVEN IF OUR HABIT FEELS RIGHT FOR US. SOME PLACES TIGHTEN, SOME SLACKEN, SOME LENGTHEN, SOME SHORTEN.

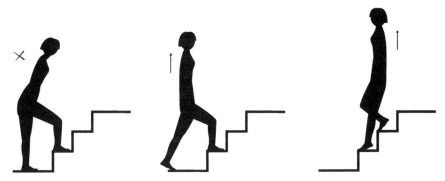

The vertical axis is efficient whether going upstairs or down

If the head wants to thrust forward we can draw it in a little, or if it tends to tilt back we can ease the chin forwards and slightly down. The long and strong spine supporting us needs its natural curves, but with no prominent kinks or exaggerations.

Make friends with gravity! See those lines of gravitational force as supportive, not oppressive. If we imagine gravity as a heavy load on our head and shoulders and life itself as a heavy burden too, we are bound to compress ourselves and bend under the strain of it all. Gravity is the basis of our posture and certainly not our enemy because we have evolved within its restraints. In the language of mechanics, it loads the very springs that activate our movement, so although this seems paradoxical it is also the source of our ability to extend upwards. If we take this image to the B/M/S entity, we notice that in other areas of life, too, it is often an apparently downward pressure that turns out to be the source of our ability to extend in other ways.

Gravity can be our friend in more than one way. Some of the exercises use the body's weight to exert a pressure that massages a joint from within. Others use the weight of a limb to produce a resisting force against which we can work to tone and strengthen some of our muscles.

Don't Try Too Hard!

Postural adjustments should never be forced. We feel wrong if we try too hard or make big alignment corrections all at once. Our posture seems to have its own ideas, often distorted by an assortment of individual habits. If we know we need to change, we should keep this alignment picture in mind, make small adjustments only, and let the improvements come slowly as the body appreciates the changes.

Increasing awareness, both from observation and from inner kinaesthetic sensing, is always self correcting. Once started, growing awareness continues to make improvements. Postural rules are useful as an outline but are much less important than good images to aim for.

The main purpose of all the loosening and gentle stretching and the relaxation exercises of this programme is to encourage the suppleness and flexibility necessary for good alignment. If we stay stiff in our joints and muscles we can never get rid of the habits of holding on too tightly and so misaligning our head, body and legs.

The positive mental inner picture of the sheer practical sense and efficiency of balanced vertical line is very important. When we do take a good look at uprightness and appreciate that it is natural and desirable and has psychological and spiritual aspects, too, we find ourselves much more willing to do a few easy exercises to allow it to return.

Proprioception and the Anti-Gravity System

Proprioception is the name of the process by which the body adjusts its balance through a nervous system millions of years old. It uses signals from wherever the muscles sense pressure, at the main points of support and at all the joints. It also uses information about balance provided by a sensitive system in the ear, and visual information collected at the same time.

As soon as we stand on our feet on firm ground – an animal would explore the ground tentatively for firmness if in doubt, and choose another spot if need be – the little muscles between the metatarsals of the feet spread as they sense the pressure of weight on them. Then instant messages flash to the spinal chord and trigger an elaborate system of support.

If we skew our feet or put our weight on an inner or outer edge disproportionately, or let ankles, knees and hips stiffen, we lose the directness of the sensory information we need. The anti-gravity muscle reflexes work automatically from all this information and adjust our balance and movement continuously. We have little control over this system but we can consciously check how we are using it from time to time, notice our feet as supporters, and try to provide the conditions it needs to work best.

Civilised life has myriads of ways of damping down this primary sensory information or deflecting our attention away from it. We like luxury and laziness and rate comfort very highly. We don't always maintain the alertness that animals have naturally, because we no longer need it for survival all the time. We don't listen to the sensory information coming in. We abstract ourselves. Whenever we are just staring into space or absenting ourselves from the here and now, we are switching off some of the information that our reflexes need to work sensitively and accurately. We are holding back some vital life energy and that diminishes posture, vision and much else.

We also have useful and enjoyable trappings such as shoes, clothes, cushions, desks, vacuum cleaners, cars, bucketed chairs and seductive sofas. And, unlike animals, we can also adopt all manner of bent and skewed poses from psychological, social, cultural and other influences. Somehow we need to learn to use all of those wonderful aids and possibilities in ways that minimise bodily misuse, and need to keep shedding and avoid accumulating the tensions that upset us.

When sitting, the ischial bones at the base of the pelvis become the support points for the weights of torso and head, and sensory information about their balance is transmitted to the spine from here. Think about them as directing your weight deep into the solid seat and down through the floor to the earth's core while your head is drawn up to the top of the sky.

If we slump back on to the sacrum, or collapse into deep cushions when sitting, information about our vertical weight bearing is limited. This is fine for comfortable reclining or relaxing short term, but not for desk work, piano playing or even holding a newspaper. Exercise Section 5B contains more detailed guidance for discovering a good sitting balance.

Summing up then, the best things we can do for our proprioception system in general, and so for our alignment and efficient body use, are to stay alert, to develop a sense of light, vertically upward extension, whether standing or

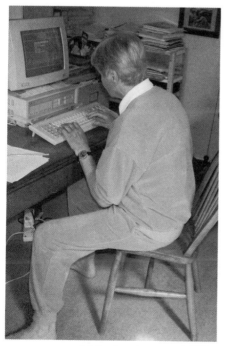 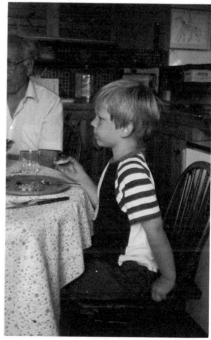

Adults often slump; small children align well without thinking about it.

sitting, and to understand that the anti-gravity system will work well automatically if we keep supple and give it good conditions and good pictures to work from. These should all, not just the exercises, be very much a part of any work we undertake to increase our personal mechanical efficiency.

Self Observation and Problem Solving

Muscles relax or release in non-stretched extension. They contract when we call on them to work for us, and release again when we let that contraction go after the job is done. The condition of restful lengthening is important as a state to return to. It is not a lazy state. The body is more alive in this condition than in a slumped or contracted one. Even the brain works more efficiently when we let go of unnecessary body tensions.

If we do not release excess tension from muscles after using them we miss out on the resting side of every equation of contract/extend, and this is tiring. Every over-contraction that we hold on to, not just in feet and legs, will work in some way to spoil the body's alignment and will use its energy wastefully. But if we are observant we can use our alignment errors as an indicator that something somewhere is needing to be released and given its chance to rest, just as we notice in other people that their misalignment often has some interesting content. Bodies can tell us a lot about the attitudes or anxieties of the owner, and sometimes reveal their occupation and interests as well.

Unfortunately, self observation has acquired a flavour of navel-watching and is often derided. We are suspicious of introspection. Narcissus was not admired for watching his own reflection. But your navel might actually need watching! Instead of taking all of our problems to an over-worked doctor and saying: "Please fix it for me!", we can often use a little intelligent self observation. Of course, we must seek professional help for serious damage or prospect of disease, but for a minor injury our own experience always has a lot of information in it and can sometimes lead us to great discoveries. Our chance reflection in a mirror or shop window or even a shadow on the wall can tell us quite a lot.

My personal bodily history contains an average, or perhaps above average, quota of accidents and enthusiastic misuse. Like many people I have had great help from doctors and also from teachers, especially of the Alexander technique. But I use the information I get from observation more and more.

Sometimes after gardening, or when tired after extra strenuous hill walking, my back aches and I can feel rather dispirited about it. But once I see my shadow or my reflection in that pulled down state it alerts me. I can lie down flat with my knees up to give my spine a rest. I can loosen up with gentle exercises. I can cheer up my spirits and enjoy whatever I am doing, because being gloomy only pulls me further down. Quite soon the pain and stiffness ease. I am not quoting this personal experience as a guaranteed cure for all backache, but for the value of the chance observation and the useful information it contains and the fact that we are able to help ourselves when we have learnt what works best for us.

In investigating your own mechanics, do tackle alignment problems with all the gentleness you would give to a child after an injury! This is not a matter of wrenching the neck into line or throwing your chest out or stretching muscles until they tear. It is a matter for quiet assessment and questioning first.

Any personal adjustment, whether of body, mind or spirit needs to be approached carefully. Experimentally yes, but not too critically and always very kindly. Do some loosening exercises where a stiffness holds you back, or some toning exercises for too much slackness. Use the visualisation processes if you suspect that the negative tensions come from your mind, or do something actively positive directed by your spirit. Better still, use all three and start to get into the way of using the whole B/M/S team together in the service of your fitness, including alignment.

Like children and most adults, bodies, minds and spirits all love to contribute when they feel noticed and know that they belong and are appreciated. Let your body, mind and spirit act as if they belong together in one supportive B/M/S team. Appreciate them! Give them good conditions! Give them sensible exercises. Encourage them to work together and exercise and stretch them all just a little! Awareness will increase on all fronts. Proprioception will wake up. And alignment will show noticeable benefits from this holistic cooperation and acknowledgement.

Nature is not a villain but she is practical. The adaptations she makes are always very practical ones. Usually they take into account the direction in which we seem to be heading. ("She doesn't seem to need those abdominals! I can save effort there.") If we use our own good sense to move towards a better alignment, Nature will rejoice in our return to naturalness with no recriminations, and will respond with restored good working.

Since we want our personal alignment adjustments as well as our whole lives to be in the direction of improvement rather than increasing collapse, and towards expanding life's quality and options not closing them down, it is in the direction of extension, uprightness and openness that we need to exercise and for an all over flexibility that can make those qualities possible.

We can cultivate an anti-gravity sense that works for us in every part, with its parallels for mind and spirit too. Our ability to take a positive direction is already there, powered by the pressures and challenges of our lives as much as by gravity. It is in full working order and only waiting for us to respect and use it.

EXERCISE SECTION 1

Basic Body Work

Equipment

1: A 1in thick foam mat or a folded blanket.

2: A small cushion or foam pad, 1in to 2in thick.

3: Two food tins of about 1lb to use as weights for upper body exercises. Don't try to use heavier weights at first but after a time you could graduate to plastic-coated dumbbells of 2lb to 3lb, no more.

4: A chair for occasional support.

Space

Find a space, preferably carpeted, not too cold, with room to stretch and move around. Allow room to extend the arms widely and above the head, too, standing or lying. Create a right-brain-friendly space that you can enjoy. This is a place for creating positive well-being, not just a workshop for running repairs.

Clothes

Wear loose, light clothes in warm weather, a warm track suit in colder weather. Bare feet are best for all the exercises. If you prefer to wear shoes, use the lightest possible ones and take them off for the feet and ankle exercises. For foot warmth, use cotton socks preferably. Nylon tights are often too restrictive for maximum freedom.

Sequence

Although there are millions of exercises we can do, and many more with which I would vary a teaching programme, this warm-up sequence has been pared to a practical minimum. If you stay within the guidelines, by all means add to it from your own favourites, but it is best not to shorten it.

Not every exercise is illustrated. It is unnecessary to show you how to shrug your shoulders, for example. But each exercise is fully described and wherever a picture can be a real help you will find one close to the written description.

After these warm-ups, which start by working from top to toe, the exercises of the later sections become more specialised. The order, in the more detailed sections that follow, is from the feet and ankles upwards. If you decide to work right through, this is a good order to choose.

If you select, do remember that tensions are rarely only localised. If, for example, you know your shoulders need loosening up it is certainly good to give them special attention. But other tightnesses, in the wrists or pelvis or even ankles, for example, can be contributing to that shoulder tension. The body operates as an integrated structure, an organic whole. Aim to maintain a balance of work at most sessions, even if time is short.

As you become familiar with the exercises and the principles underlying them, and more fully acquainted with your personal needs, you will be able to construct your own best workout.

There is no danger in this work of producing a conspicuously different way of moving. You are encouraging your own unique body to become freer in movement so that its automatic systems of balance are freed to work for you effectively. It will be you, your distinctive self, who becomes more poised, feels more alive and more expressively you, not an inappropriate stereotype dictated for you.

How Much Time?

Don't be seduced by books and articles that suggest you can make noticeable changes to your fitness in five minutes a day of one magical exercise! We cannot do this. Our fitness stays related to our current, general, overall, everyday body usage. If this is perfect and our life very active, we need less time for formal exercise, but most of us need at least 15 to 20 minutes daily to make up for missing suppleness, and we benefit from several longer periods within a week.

Regular exercises can indeed work wonders. But this only happens if that exercise is also gently educating our bodies to be more aware and to use their natural suppleness well. Only then can we make a significant long-term difference. Nevertheless it is true that every little helps.

It is also true that an exercise done awarely for a particular purpose, and with its benefits noticed appreciatively afterwards, has longer lasting effects than one done sketchily and thoughtlessly.

Weigh up for yourself how active you are and how well you use your body, and what demands you make of it. These overlapping considerations will help to determine how much exercise you need, considering your own unique life style. Be open to the supreme worthwhileness of gradually releasing old restrictions and liberating all your movements.

All the exercises are simple to do and to learn. To make a noticeable impact on everyday fitness, I recommend:

❑ At least 15 minutes every morning from the basics of this section, preferably doing them all.

❑ Some deliberate daily practice during ordinary activities. For example, choose to stand well for a few minutes, sit well right through a concert, meal or television programme, or lie well for a period of real relaxation. Experiment with moving more awarely and more lightly in several mundane tasks during the day, such as reaching to open a door or to high or low cupboards, ironing or preparing food.

❏ Later each day, do 10 minutes of specialised exercises for a particular area of your personal needs. Choose some stretches or other quite different exercises from the later sections of the programme to maintain a balance of work.

❏ I have not included exercises for strength or stamina or cardio vascular work. During the week, fit in at least three periods of half an hour of your favourite sport, aerobics, recreational walking or swimming. Gradually increase these times if possible. You will soon want to do so as you come to enjoy the growing feeling of energy, lightness and suppleness.

❏ Sometimes take a full hour or 1½ hours, as you would in a regular exercise class, and cover all the exercises in full. Never push against the clock. Take time to give each one its full value and to notice what it is doing for you.

These are NOT PHYSICAL JERKS! In each exercise remember to lengthen and lighten upwards. Try using the Oriental image of a flying kite lifting the crown of your head towards the sky while your feet are firmly grounded. And enjoy the fact that in making this a regular daily workout you are returning your whole body to the flexibility that is natural to it.

The Warm-up Exercises

1: Breathing

There are eight full breaths in this cycle. Take them slowly and fully but don't over-breathe! It is a good way to start. You only have to stand up and begin! The movements stimulate a demand for more oxygen by using all four limbs as well as the rib cage. It is not an iron cage, by the way. Your rib cage is flexible and should be allowed to expand in width and depth without any forcing. Feel that the whole torso opens to accept a full breath and then gently expels all its air. As you breathe in, abdomen, ribs, back and upper back all expand. And the out breath starts also in the abdominal area and then goes from the ribcage, chest and back as well. The cycle can be repeated, but make pauses, and stop if you feel you have done enough with just one cycle of eight breaths.

First two breaths

Stand with the feet a few inches apart, evenly weighted, the body relaxed and lengthening up. Release any neck tension. Chin approximately level.

Breathe in, lifting the arms lightly up in front, palms up, to shoulder level. Let one lead slightly, to avoid a tight symmetry in the movements (Figure 1.1).

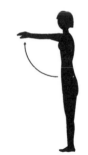

Figure 1.1

At the end of the in-breath, turn the hands palms down, and as you breathe out, send the knees forwards and out and let the out breath take you down into a squat. Heels rise, or may be kept on the floor, as you descend as far as feels comfortable (Figure 1.2).

Turn palms up and use the second in-breath to lift you to the position of Figure 1.1 again, and the second out-breath to take you down again.

Second two breaths

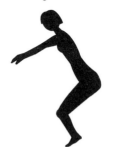

Figure 1.2

Breathe in and rise up from the squatting position, lifting the arms softly out to the sides this time, palms open and up as the breath lifts you up, (Figure 1.3), palms over and down and as you breathe out and lower the body to squat again (Figure 1.4). Repeat this movement.

Third two breaths

Breathe in, rising up with the hands forward again, then out as you lower arms and body – and do this twice.

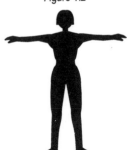

Figure 1.3

Seventh and eighth breaths

Repeat the lift with widespread arms, and the squatting as before. But for the eighth and last full breath of the sequence, rise up, floating the arms out to shoulder level, and then stay standing and lower your arms softly to your sides as you breathe out.

Pause between cycles and then repeat this cycle once or perhaps twice. The second and third

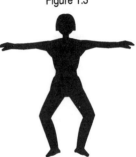

Figure 1.4

cycles can be a little slower and fuller than the first, but avoid arching back or taking hugely extravagant breaths. And if you are just beginning to exercise, eight full breaths are enough.

2: Neck and face

Circle the head quite slowly, clockwise several times and then anti-clockwise. Yawn as you do this. Make bigger and bigger yawns as the circles grow bigger. They release tension that might be there in jaw, face and eye muscles. Don't force these circles. Start very small. Let the shoulders and spine join in as you make bigger circles. Really big noisy yawns can trigger some eye watering to brighten the eyes as well, and will top up the vital oxygen supply to body and brain.

Follow the circles with three or four gentle falls of the neck, to the right and the left and forwards and back. Keep the neck lengthening up. As your head falls to the right, slide your right hand down the side of the right thigh so that the whole spine joins in. With all the falls, pause after the first, breathe in and then go a little further on the out-breath, and return slowly. Repeat for the left (Figure 1.5).

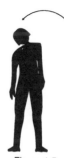

Figure 1.5

As the head falls forwards, let the wide shoulders and just the upper spine round down slightly.

As the head falls back, lengthen your front all the way up from the solar plexus to the throat without shortening the neck. Expand the rib cage and widen across the upper chest too, leaning back a little. Again feel the cervical spine to be just a part of the length of the whole spine, not a separate entity, as it lengthens and curves gently back (Figure 1.6).

You will feel taller, the abdominals firmer, too, after these head rolls and falls if you have done them slowly and fully. You might feel shorter and more compressed if you hunched the neck or tried to do the various falls only for the neck separately from the spine.

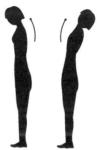

Figure 1.6

3: Shoulder shrugs and waves

Stand with feet apart at first, evenly weighted, the whole body upright and lengthening up. See that you are not leaning, slumping forwards, arching back or tightening anything.

Circle the right shoulder back four times, loosely and slowly. Repeat with the left shoulder.

Circle each shoulder forwards in turn, four times.

Now take a small forward step on the left foot, and try the right shoulder circles with a little more involvement of the rest of the body. This will give more rib cage movement than when the torso was still. Experiment with changing the weight from front to back foot and then from back to front while circling the right shoulder, using some momentum from the foot that is weighted.

Circle the left shoulder with this same stance. Try all possible variations.

Then change to the right foot forward, and again do both forward and back shoulder circles with both forward and backward movements of the body, first with the left shoulder and then with the right.

Lastly, some big arm circles – underarm first. With the left foot forward, carry your weight over that foot and take the right arm forwards across you. Turn the palm out and let the hand sweep a big circle, slowly, from front to back, transferring your weight to the back foot and watching the hand.

Head and body turn together with the leading movement of hand and arm. At the fullest extent, wave to an imagined friend far behind you. Complete the circle, slowly bringing the arm round to your side and forward and your weight over the front foot again.

Repeat twice and then for the left arm, with the right foot forward. Think about the improved safety you gain when driving as you keep this big rotational freedom alive in arm, shoulder, mobile ribs and waist.

Note that much of the momentum for this underarm swing comes from the forward weighted foot.

Follow these underarm circles with three overarm ones. Start this reverse action with the weight over the back foot, right knee bent, torso turned to the right, the right arm hanging beside you. The action is like that of a cricket bowler, the rear foot again supplying much of the energy of the big circular swing of the arm as your weight transfers to the front foot.

4: Arm, hand and wrist stretching and loosening

Stand with the feet apart and move your weight across to the right side. Lean out and extend the right arm, then rotate it, little finger up, then right round to stretch the thumb up. The rotation goes from fingers to wrist, elbow and right into the shoulder. Repeat (Figure 1.7). Move your weight across to the left and repeat for the left arm. Watch the hand movement each time.

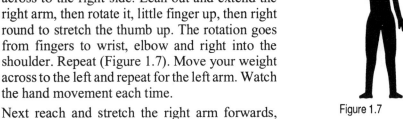

Figure 1.7

Next reach and stretch the right arm forwards, palm down. Stretch the fingers up, as if stopping traffic, pushing the wrist straight ahead. Then bend the hand down from the wrist, stretching the back of the wrist. Repeat both stretches and repeat for the left arm..

After these stretches, lean out to one side, let the arm fall loosely from the shoulder and gently shake the hand to loosen thumb, fingers, the wrist, elbow and shoulder joints, shifting your attention into these areas one by one. Repeat for the other arm.

For a glimpse of the importance of an upright stance and open shoulders for arm freedom, try some small variations of body position for simple arm raising. Slouch the whole body first – round the shoulders in and raise the arms forwards. Now lower them, return to a balanced upright, extend the shoulder widely out and lift the arms forwards again. Repeat the exercise seeing what you can notice about the movements.

If you have not noticed a much lighter action from the upright, open stance, exaggerate the slouch more and when upright lighten up more. (Its not a sergeant major uprightness that is wanted.) All arm movements can become wonderfully light when the spine is well aligned, shoulders wide, upper chest high and open, back not arched or slumped. Try just floating them up, forwards, to the sides, above the head, everywhere. The difference you notice from practising this exercise regularly can be very useful to you when driving, working at a bench or sink, or reading a book.

Raise both arms forward lightly, one after the other, and do some free ballet, piano or typing movements, or imagine holding a newspaper.

Lastly raise both hands in front of the chest and shake them freely but not fiercely. Shake them up and down, side to side and round and round, both ways, freeing up all the possibilities of the complex wrist joint. Then alternately tighten into fists and extend the whole hand to stretch it.

5: Loose arm swings

With the feet well apart, rotate the upper body loosely from the waist, to the right and then the left. Let the arms and whole body relax. Feel like a child in

the playground, letting the world go by. As you swing, the arms flail round of themselves, following the body's momentum and wrapping round the waist. Your weight travels from one foot to the other, the unweighted foot pivoting on the toe.

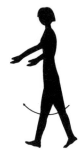

Watch your horizon all the way round. Feel like a rotating pendulum with wide-eyed vision.

It is relaxing to continue this loosening exercise for many cycles, but choose to stop when you feel that you have had a sufficient loosening up time (Figure 1.8).

Figure 1.8

6: Side stretches

Raise the right arm quite softly and roundly above the head, either close past your chest and face, or sweeping round widely to the side. This avoids involving and, perhaps, kinking the back. Don't let the torso twist round. The arches of both pelvis and ribcage, although you are now going to stretch the gap between them, stay in the same vertical plane. Imagine them sandwiched between two big sheets of plate glass.

Bring the left hand up and back to spread along the middle back to help you to notice and remove any excess arching of the spine. Then tilt over to the left side and when nicely stretched, breathe out and then slowly take two full breaths (Figure 1.9).

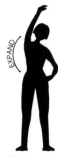

The right side of the rib cage will expand and feel an extra stretch as you breathe into it, and your lungs will find extra room to expand in. After the first breath, increase the angle of tilt so that the second full breath is even bigger.

Figure 1.9

Return to upright again. Repeat for the left side with the same attention to leaving the torso unarched and not rotated.

7: Spinal stretch

With fists pummelling into the mid-back, lengthen and lean back from the waist, not centrally at first but via small rotating movements from side to side. Your back will shorten and the front lengthen (Figure 1.10).

Return to the balanced lengthened upright position.

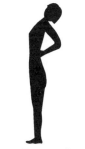

Figure 1.10

Place the hands now on the front of the upper thighs, to support the back ready to curl forwards (Figure 1.11).

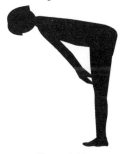

Lengthen again, tip the head forwards on its high pivot first and, leaning forwards, curl the spine down, sliding the hand support down to the knees. Then remove the hands and let the weight of your head carry you down until you hang loosely (Figure 1.12).

Figure 1.11

Swing loosely for a few moments as your spine gently stretches. Uncurl slowly. Then repeat the backward and forward stretches once.

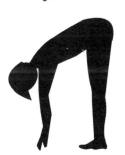

Figure 1.12

8: Pelvic circles

With feet wide apart, place hands firmly on the sides of the pelvis and circle the hips around. Push them to one side and then to the back, the other side, and round to the front, pressing the pelvis forwards like a belly dancer. Circle a few times one way and then the other (Figure 1.13).

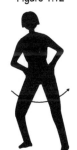

Figure 1.13

9: Knee circles

With feet a few inches apart and heels on the ground, lengthen up, and then send the knees forward to lower the spine a little way vertically. Next release the hips to go back and fold at hip level. Lastly, place a hand just above each knee and relax into a partial squat (Figure 1.14).

Pressing down on the knees with your hands, circle them a few times in each direction. Don't rise, but go into the next exercise from this position.

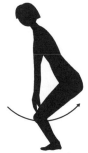

Figure 1.14

10: Ankle weighting

Sill in a partial squat, heels on the floor, relax the lower back, hips, knees and ankles and press down lightly to compress the ankle joints a little further than they usually go. Then transfer your weight to one ankle, springing it a little, and then to the other. Come back to standing and shake each leg loosely, all the way from the ankle to the hip joint.

Take a few moments to walk about after this exercise.

Having loosened up from top to toe, the last exercises of this basic sequence are for coordination and for posture.

11: Coordination cross-overs

These give the whole body some nice free movements and energise the brain too. They use the linkages between the brain hemispheres and encourage more active cooperation between them. They are very simple. If you have problems with coordination, take them slowly, do them often and look forward to steady improvement.

(i) Slapping the opposite knee

Raise the left knee and bring the lightly cupped right hand across to meet it. Change and cross left hand to right knee. Keep your attention on the meeting of these opposite limbs. Don't go too fast. Continue for at least 12 movements.

(ii) High rise

Lift the left knee and raise your right arm high above the head, neck free, head lightly forward, back not arched. Alternate this action for several cycles. After some practice, vary the use of the eyes. Look up for three counts, down for three, then to one side and then the other for three counts each (Figure 1.15).

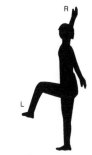

Figure 1.15

(iii) Heel kicks

Lift the left heel behind you and slap it with the right hand (Figure 1.16). Repeat with the right heel and the left hand. Continue for 10 or more kicks.

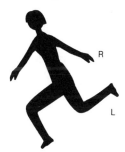

Figure 1.16

(iv) Diagonal stretches

Extend the right hand high up, a little forward, and out to your right side with the left foot diagonally back and out to the left, stretching into these opposite extremities (Figure 1.17).

Avoid tilting the head back or arching the back. If it helps you, take the free hand behind you to check that the back does not arch. Repeat these alternating movements for 5 to 10 cycles

There are more of these coordination movements in Section 11. Vary them in your regular work-out. They refresh the brain, the vision and other senses and loosen up and invigorate the body.

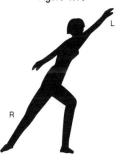

Figure 1.17

12: Maximum bi-pedal range

Sky-reaching and Squats

(i) Start with the feet shoulder width apart.

With an open and easy swing, turn to your right and swing both arms lightly across to the right side without straining. Let the unweighted left foot turn a little with the movement (Figure 1.18). Flexing ankles and knees, swing across to the left.

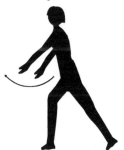

Figure 1.18

Continue these movements, gradually extending into an upward and backward turn and reach, and lowering further through the central position. As you widen the stance, let the following foot turn in the direction of the arms until you are turning as far as you can. Follow the hands with your eyes until you are looking up to an imagined moon high above and behind you, and touching the floor in front on the way across between the rotations (Figures1.19 and 1.20). After three or four big swings, finish in the low central position.

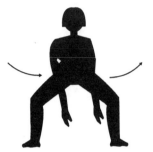

Figure 1.19

(ii) Stay in the wide, low squatting position and explore your reach in all directions (Figure 1.21). Imagine you are placing or picking up objects on low shelves or on the floor.

(iii) Stand with feet apart, body upright, and then walk around imagining you are placing things on high and low shelves. Move lightly and expansively.

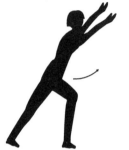

Figure 1.20

Having stretched a little further, the body gets interested in that extra scope. It starts to enjoy using a bigger range, and so will your mind and spirit.

13: The level head

You need a full length mirror for this exercise, or a partner to hold your head while you turn your body.

(i) Stand upright but relaxed, looking ahead at your eyes in the mirror. See that they are level or allow your partner's hold to keep them level (Figure 1.22).

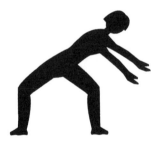

Figure 1.21

(ii) Keep eye contact with yourself if using a mirror, and take small steps to rotate the body at least a right angle and further round if easy. Check all the time that your eyes stay level and the body upright.

(iii) Without a pause, rotate right back again with little steps, and round to the other side. Keep up a continuous flow of movement from side to side,

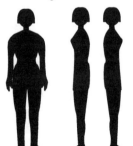

Figure 1.22

the eyes remaining level all the time and small steps turning your upright body underneath the head.

This exercise is partly for observation of your own uprightness. Any torso leaning or head thrusting shows up and can be noticed and thought about and perhaps corrected little by little – never criticised! It also lengthens the spine as it corkscrews around like a spiral staircase, and it frees the neck. After four or five rotations, you should feel much better aligned.

Everyday Reminders

In everyday activities, return to the fluidity of these exercises and make movements around home or office or on country walks more interesting and more lively. Giving and taking, placing or dusting, even opening a door, all work much better when the body extends as a whole and takes pleasure in the movement itself.

Let the direction of the whole body, feet, pelvis, torso, hands and eyes be wholehearted. Face in the direction of the movement you intend to make. Enjoy transferring your weight from foot to foot without sinking into the hip joint. And use odd moments to loosen and stretch ankles, wrists, arms, spine, shoulders etc., as in these warm-ups. They are all meant as reminders and re-educators, as well as for specific loosening and warming-up.

Even if these are the only exercises you use from this book, as you grow familiar with them you will find them more and more valuable. Fitness cannot really be *banked*. We only keep our faculties by using them regularly and using them well. But a nice fact emerges with regular practice. The exercises continue to teach you how to do them well and how to use your body well.

Don't worry if early attempts seem muddled or inaccurate. Persist with them and keep discovering new things about them and yourself and about the organic whole that your body is. The warm-up sequence is an ABC of movement that illuminates the B/M/S wholeness, too, in subtle ways. It makes a very valuable contribution to our general fitness.

Air Travel Exercises

Exercises from this warming up group can be adapted to use as an antidote to the prolonged sitting of long journeys. Perhaps warn your neighbour! Some of them can be done seated, but it would be better to claim a space in the aisle and do them as fully as possible. Try especially to use the squatting movements, as in the breathing and low reaching exercises, and the stretches for the upper body, for front, back and sides. These will work those big leg muscles and the arms and rib cage in a way that helps with the circulation after such a long time sitting.

EXERCISE SECTION 2

Feet and Ankles

Introduction

Whenever you have time, include these exercises in the general loosening and stretching programme of the everyday workout.

If you ever wonder if they are worthwhile, take a look around at some older people who do not take much exercise and notice how posture, agility and even safety are restricted when feet and ankles lose their resilience. Don't use that as negative motivation. Just notice that you have a positive opportunity to do better than that by staying supple.

Props: A chair to hold lightly for balance. A wooden block to stand on, or a step, or the top or bottom of a staircase with handrail.

Footwear: Bare feet or comfortable cotton socks.

The Exercises

1: Toe presses

Curl the big toe under and press down on it, stretching the muscles and loosening the small joints in the arch of the foot. Apply pressure gently, but use enough to feel a good stretch (Figure 2.1).

Press the other way (Figure 2.2).

Repeat these movements several times.

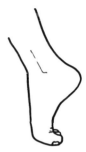

Figure 2.1

2: Arch presses

As 1, but do the same actions in different directions, all the way around a circle. Turn the knee out for arch presses diagonally forward and then to the side. Turn the knee in as you reach the back diagonal. Finish with the foot well behind you, pressing to stretch the whole front length of the instep. Between stretches reverse the pressure – as Figure 2.2 – from time to time. Repeat for the other foot.

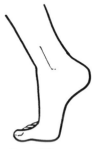

Figure 2.2

3: Ankle kicks

Do 8 or 10 loose little kicks forwards, lightly but firmly to loosen the ankle joint. Let the forward swing of your foot follow the natural line of the hip swing, just outside the mid-line.

Then direct the kick out a little, then all the way round in a circle, until kicking behind you.
Repeat for the other ankle.

4: Ankle circling

Extend one leg diagonally forward and circle the foot around the ankle six times in one direction and six the other way. Repeat for the other leg (Figure 2.3).

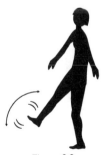

Now raise the foot behind you and circle it six times in each direction. Repeat both movements for the other foot (Figure 2.4). Then shake each leg softly and loosely all the way from hip to knees, ankle and foot.

Figure 2.3

5: Weighting the foot and ankle

(a) Step forward with one foot and take your weight forward over the ankle. Lower the pelvis, with sitting bones down as if sitting, and keep your torso upright. Don't sink the upper body into the pelvis. Try to keep your length all the way up from the hip, and stay open right across pelvis and shoulders.

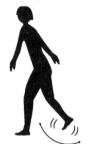

Figure 2.4

Use your natural springiness and the hinges of the ankle and knee to press down just a little and lift up vertically, several times, putting more pressure on the ankle than you usually do. Spring very lightly up and down, just enough to feel the pressure, and a little release, in the ankle (Figure 2.5).

Don't lock the neck. If it stays free your head will jog very slightly with the spring.

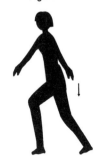

Figure 2.5

(b) Next take your weight over the back foot. With the foot and knee turned out, *sit* your weight back and spring up and down a little, as before, the torso vertical and not sunk into the hip. The weight of your body will be pressing down on the ankle, flexing the knee without compressing the hip joint. Spring enough to stress the ankle a little, but avoid jarring bounces (Figure 2.6).

Repeat (a) and (b) then repeat with the other foot forward.

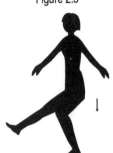

Figure 2.6

Next swing freely from (a) to (b) with arms swinging loosely forwards and back. Weight each foot fully in turn, slightly lifting the unweighted one. Exchange feet positions after about 10 swings.

(c) Stand upright, the feet a few inches apart, holding a chair or other support. Lengthening up, rise on to tip-toes and back again, 10 times. Keep upright and open, balanced vertically above the points of support. Do this 10 times (Figure 2.7).

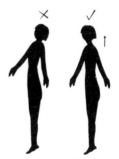

Figure 2.7

Transfer most of your weight to the right foot and repeat the tip-toe rises and falls with the right ankle weighted. Do six. Repeat for the left foot.

An easy mistake is to begin the tip-toe exercises with a forward and upward thrust of the chest, anticipating the vertical lift. Instead, just drop the chin very slightly and lean a little forwards from the ankles. You can then rise in a nice vertical line without that alignment distortion.

(d) Stand on a step or a wooden block, with the heels free, the front of the foot arch resting along the edge of the step. Use hand support. Repeat tip-toe rises of (c) from this position, first with both feet sharing your weight, and then one at a time. Lower the heel below the level of the step before lifting up on to the toes each time (Figure 2.8).

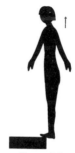

Figure 2.8

(e) On the floor again, rise on tip toes, feet a little apart. Still lengthening up to the crown of the head, let your knees go forwards and lower the whole body into an upright and balanced squat (Figure 2.9). To return to standing on tip toes, while the left hand supports you, lean forwards, touch the floor with fingertips of the right hand and push up lightly. Your leg reflexes will lift you up. Repeat four times.

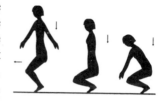

Figure 2.9

Benefits

These exercises make a big difference to agility, springiness, posture and balance. You can safely look forward to being 90 if you persist with them.

All weight-bearing exercises also contribute to the way the bones use and store calcium, so these will also help to fend off osteoporosis, a hazard especially for women after middle age.

As you exercise, Nature notices – "this person seems to need strength in the structure just here" – and summons supplies of the necessary minerals, oxygen and nutrients to the places you exercised.

If the improved strength and agility encourages you to enjoy a new sport or take daily walks and become more active generally as well, this particular benefit to the bones themselves is enormously enhanced. Table tennis, which can be played even by the elderly is a very good non-stressful exercise for feet, ankles, backs too, and wonderful for general agility.

Everyday Reminders

Because shoes restrict our feet for many hours of every day, aim to take off your shoes at home quite often.

Avoid standing motionless for long. Move your weight around. Use the whole foot, right to the toes. Notice the ball of the foot in action as you walk.

Stretch and rotate the ankles sometimes, and use your ankle power whenever reaching, stretching or squatting, to extend both height and depth and reach.

These exercises can be fitted into quite small cracks in the time table. Before putting on shoes in the morning, or when changing to different ones, do a few toe presses while the feet are free. But ankle kicks and circles and weighting and squats can easily be done at odd moments, even with shoes on.

EXERCISE SECTION 3

Legs

The Exercises

Introduction

This is a very valuable group of exercises that make a positive difference to posture and freedom of movement.

Stretches come first and should be done slowly, never suddenly, and always preceded by warming up. Muscles take a sudden stretch as a danger signal and react by holding on tight. If the stretch is then forced, as in an accident or the sudden emergency of many sports injury situations, both muscle fibres and connective tissue between them may tear.

If your exercise demand is gentle and sustained, the muscles you are working on release that panic reflex and will gently lengthen. A good stretch feels good. Extend gently before each stretch, preparing the muscles to take the strain.

After stretches come exercises to tone up and strengthen the muscles of the leg and its links with the pelvis and lower back, then a programme to train the three leg hinges to work together.

Lastly, linking with the whole body, we work with the full range of side to side movement again, as introduced in the warm-up group of Section 1.

The Exercises

Props: Use a chair for support, placed firmly beside a wall. For Exercise 3, face the lower steps of a staircase, and for 4c use an exercise bench or a space at the top of the stairs from which to lower the legs while lying.

1: Calf stretch

Use both hands on the back of the chair or, better still, against a wall bar or strong newell post or very firm table top. Take a comfortable step back with the right leg to stretch the big calf muscle and Achilles tendon, pressing the heel away and down. Extend gently first, then stretch slowly, adjusting your weight to give a strong but not a forced stretch. Hold for from 10 to 20 seconds as tensions slowly release (Figure 3.1).

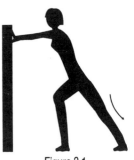

Figure 3.1

Repeat this exercise with the heel lifted and the right knee bent. The stretch will now reach the lower muscles between ankle and calf (Figure 3.1a).

Repeat for the left leg, then repeat both stretches

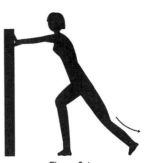

Figure 3.1a

for each leg, turning the direction of the foot a little
so that different muscle fibres will be involved.

Variation 1:

Repeat with hands high up and flat against a wall,
to include a nice whole-body stretch. Keep your
head between the arms and avoid arching the back.
Aim for one long line (Figure 3.1b).

Variation 2:

With strong table support at about hip or waist
level, rise on alternate feet, walking on the spot
without lifting the toes. Don't just lift the heel but

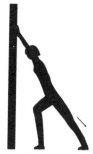

Figure 3.1b

put all your weight on one foot first, rise up on the toes, and then transfer to
the other, with an *up and over* lift, carrying the weight across as in walking.
Keep the shoulder line close to the support and relax the shoulders down.
Shoulders and arms are going to take more and more weight as you move the
feet back.

Step back, keeping chest and shoulders forward,
and repeat the walking movements for five or six
more steps, slowly, at this bigger distance.

Step back again and repeat. Extend the heel right
back towards the floor during these very inclined
stretches, and pause at each one for a good stretch.

As the lower calf muscles and tendons become
gently stretched, this exercise can be done as a
continuous backwards and forwards walk, slowly
increasing the angle of lean from the ankles as you
go back. Pressure on the arms is relieved as you
move forwards in this more mobile version, but

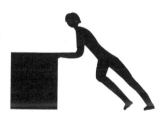

Figure 3.1c

practice should be done gently and slowly with all of them (Figure 3.1c).

2: Quadriceps stretch

Lift the right knee forward and grasp the right
ankle. Draw it up behind you. Lower the sitting
bones towards the floor (Figure 3.2). The pelvis
needs to be vertically aligned, the torso long, the
back not arched, head level.

Lift the arm loosely, without thrusting out the
chest or kinking the back, and balance with it
rounded above your head. If balancing is difficult,
this hand should be used for support (Figure 3.3).

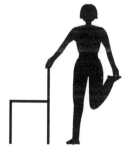

Fiugure 3.2

Breathe in, lengthening the whole body upwards and widening at shoulder level. On the out breath, pull the foot closer to your seat and lengthen down the right thigh into the knee to increase the stretch.

Hold the stretch for a count of 6 to 10.

Breathe in and lengthen up again, and repeat the two-way stretch and the hold while breathing out. Then release the foot and relax.

Repeat for the left leg, and for each leg again.

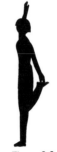

Figure 3.3

Benefits: As with all the muscle stretches, this exercise improves the circulation and removes stagnant waste chemicals. It is good after sitting for long periods, and before, during, and after strenuous sports such as hill walking, tennis or jogging, because the quadriceps tighten from sustained and strenuous use as well as from under-use.

3: Hamstring stretches

(a) One leg at a time
Preparation

Stand facing the lower steps of a staircase. Raise the right foot to rest its heel on the first or second stair. Adjust the left leg to be a strong vertical support, with the foot evenly weighted, body balanced uprightly above the foot (Figure 3.4).

Check with your hands at the hips that the hip line is parallel to the steps. There is a temptation in this exercise to swing the hip out and rotate the body as you reach forwards, in an effort to lean further.

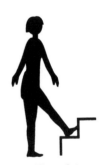

Figure 3.4

To keep the back from rounding over, take your hands behind your back, lengthen up out of the pelvis, open up the upper chest and incline the torso forwards (Figure 3.5).

Take the hands down to the front fold line of the hips and incline a little further. Keep the spine extended. To avoid rounding the back or contracting your neck into the shoulders, think about shoulders being down and out, the chin slightly in, and all the neck vertebrae lengthening headwards. Don't even think about trying to flex fur-

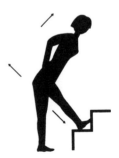

Figure 3.5

ther forward if the back rounds over, but hold this mini-stretch for six counts.

For some of us – and hamstring tightness has been a long-term problem for me – this introductory small lean may be enough for our first few attempts at this exercise. Just change the leg positions, straighten both legs, and work through the preparatory alignment details and the exploratory extension. Use the fingertips to keep the pelvis in line. Feel that you are lengthening the whole of the back of the extended right leg, the hip lengthening away from the heel.

The Main Exercise

To stretch the right leg further, if you are ready to do so:

(i) While breathing in, flex slightly more forwards from the hips. Hold for three counts. Then exhale and relax in this position (Figure 3.5a).

Steps (ii), (iii) and (iv) are only added after some regular practice with the first stage.

(ii) Breathe in again, lengthen again and flex a little further forward and down. Release the tail bones back. Hold for a few moments then relax.

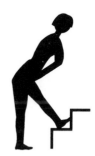

Figure 3.5a

As your flexion increases, transfer both hands to the right hip fold and press back here as if to help elongate both the body and the leg. Relax any tightness in the forward foot. It should rest lightly on the heel as the hip lengthens away from it.

(iii) With the third inhalation, see if you can go further still, and hold the stretch for 5 to 10 counts before exhaling and relaxing.

(iv) Breathe in a fourth time, take the flexion as far as you comfortably can, and hold again, for 10 counts or more. Relax as you breathe out.

Repeat this sequence for the left leg.

After regular practice, a higher step level could be used, never higher than hip level. But in my experience with general classes, there is plenty of stretch at step 2 for most people.

(b) For both legs together

The following exercises for both legs together are not unnatural if your legs are equally fit. If you know them to be different in length or fitness, stick to the previous exercise and work one leg at a time.

(i) Crouch down with the heels on or off the floor, fingers on the floor in front. Then push the bottom

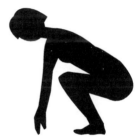

Figure 3.6a

up, to stand as an inverted V. Hold this position, sending the sitting bones high (Figure 3.6, a and b). Crouch down again and repeat.

(ii) With the feet apart and about 18in from a wall, lean the seat back to rest on the wall. Now lean forwards with the upper chest open. Hands may rest on the thighs, or fingertips back on the wall behind as you gradually increase the angle of leaning (Figure 3.7). The exercise gives more stretch with the feet closer to the wall, so adjust the gap until it feels just right for you. If you press the feet to the floor and try to send the ischial bones higher up the wall you will achieve a really good stretch for the hamstrings. Hold for several seconds at the maximum enjoyable stretch.

Figure 3.6b

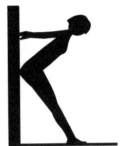

Figure 3.7

4: Stretches for inner leg, thigh and lower back

(a) Standing

Use a wide natural stride (Figure 3.8).

Turn to face the right foot and take your weight forwards on to it, bending the right knee and lifting the heel. Reach hands to the floor in front of the foot to support some of your weight and lower the body over the forward foot. Turn to face forwards and towards the floor. Feel a good stretch in the inner thigh muscles of the extended left leg (Figure 3.9). Maintain this stretch for 10 counts.

If you cannot reach a deep squat, go only as far as is comfortable and hold for a few seconds only.

Return to the wide stride, face the left foot, and repeat the exercise on that side, and once more each way.

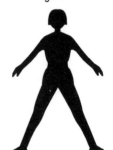

Figure 3.8

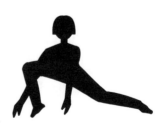

Figure 3.9

Variation

Keep both feet flat on the floor. Rest your right forearm on the right thigh and press it down on the thigh for a good stretch. Don't force the stretch. Repeat for the left side (Figure 3.10).

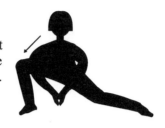

Figure 3.10

(b) Lying

Lie comfortably. Lift and extend the right leg, then flex the knee and draw it up towards the chest. Hold it firmly but not fiercely, just below the knee. Don't lift the head or round the back. Inhale, pushing your chest up towards the thigh, not pulling the thigh towards your chest. On the out breath gradually draw the knee gently closer. Inhale again, lifting chest towards thigh. Exhale, drawing the knee slightly further headwards. Do three full breaths like this, then hold for a few counts (Figure 3.11).

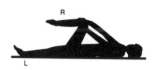

Figure 3.11

Next, retaining the upward pull, draw the knee out to your right side, holding this outward and headward stretch for about 10 counts (Figure 3.12). Keep the straight leg extended. Shoulders and head do not lift.

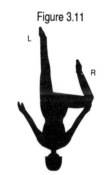

Figure 3.12

Now reach for your right foot with the left hand and bring it to the top of the left thigh and curve the free arm above your head for a nice stretch.

Gradually release the muscles and let the knee fall out. The position is similar to that of a Yoga half-lotus. Relax into this stretch and hold for 10 counts (Figure 3.13).

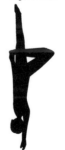

Figure 3.13

Extend the leg again before lowering it to the
floor, and then repeat all three stretches in sequence for the left leg.

(c) Lying on an exercise bench or top of a stairway

Lie with the lower back at the very edge of the
bench or the top of the stairs, both feet on the floor
(if you are on a bench), or on the second step down
the stairs. Thighs should be horizontal (Figure
3.14). Draw your right knee towards the chest and
clasp it lightly, angled out a little from the mid-
line.

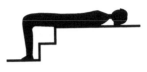

Figure 3.14

Now extend the left leg so that its weight pulls it
in a falling curve, lightly stretching the muscles
of the left thigh. Hold for 10 counts (Figure 3.15).
Relax.

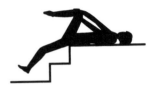

Figure 3.15

For an extra stretch, raise the left arm back along
the floor as you extend the left leg, holding this
position for 10 counts. Repeat, exchanging the leg
and arm positions (Figure 3.16). Rest with feet
side by side.

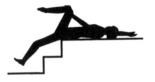

Figure 3.16

Variation for Extra Muscle Toning

Don't attempt this stronger variation if the basic
exercise gives you discomfort.

Clasp the right knee and extend the left leg.

Lift the extended leg to just above the horizontal
and circle it three times in each direction (Figure
3.17). Then raise it up for several inches, back to
horizontal again then let it relax down again (as in
Figure 3.15). Repeat the raise, lower, relax, se-

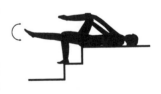

Figure 3.17

quence twice more, and then change legs. Stretch, circle, and raise and lower the other leg, again, three times in all. (Figure 3.18)

If you walk around after this exercise you should feel a noticeable extra strength in the legs and a better poise in your walk.

Benefits: As well as stretching and strengthening the muscles of the thigh and exercising the hip joint, this exercise reaches muscles within the pelvis that link the mid-back to the top of the leg-bone. Tightness in these inner muscles folds the body forwards. Stretching and toning them makes it easier to maintain a lengthened front and good vertical alignment.

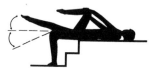

Figure 3.18

5: Using the three hinges of the legs

(a) Stand with the feet a little apart and take a natural step forward on the right foot. Transfer your weight to that foot, the knee forwards over it.

Tuck the buttocks slightly under as if sitting and spring up and down above the foot, to feel the natural reflexive action at work in ankle and knee, as in ankle weighting in Section 2 (Figure 2.5).

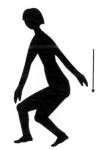

Figure 3.19

Now bring the buttocks hinge into play: Flex the ankle and knee as before, but direct your seat back, to fold at the right hip joint, and slowly lower the body further, consciously using the three hinges of ankle knee and hip all together. Extend forwards, look to the floor, and descend until your hand touches the floor outside the foot (Figure 3.19).

Keep the upper chest open. Don't round the back over or tilt the head back. Watch the floor in front.

Raise and lower the body as if picking up and putting down some imaginary object beside the foot. Repeat the up and down movements five times. As the muscles grow stronger, increase the number to 10.

Repeat on the other side.

(b) With feet apart, lengthen up, rise on to the toes, and then allow both knees to move forwards and out, lowering the body vertically, with the spine still directed up. Hinge at the hips until you are in a deep squat, heels lifted. Reach forwards as if to pick up something centrally from the floor, looking down and around this imaginary object, so that the neck stays relaxed. Explore your reach with each hand, and then with both at once, in all directions (Figure 3.20).

To stand, press on the floor in front with finger tips of both hands, helping the reflexive upward spring with a little push. Lengthen up into standing.

(c) Stand with legs more widely astride and weighted evenly. Keep the heels on the floor this time. Send both knees forward and the seat well back, folding at the hip line. Ankles, knees and hips of both legs lower you into a wide partial squat, heels still on the floor. Explore your reach from here, stretching well forwards and around, underneath you and in all directions (Figure 3.21).

(d) Stand uprightly with a wide stride. Direct the knees forwards and out. Do not send the seat back this time but lower the spine vertically, as if to sit. Keep the front long, abdominals braced, and stay in this position for several seconds or a whole minute or more. Try to release knee, calf and thigh tensions.

This position is like that of the *horse* position that martial arts practitioners use for strengthening the legs. It can be shallow or deep. It is important to stay upright and not to sink the torso into the pelvis or to let the neck tighten back. Feel your weight spreading across the balls of the feet and into the heels. Imagine you are breathing through the feet!

The head should float, chin horizontal, eyes to the horizon, the crown as if suspended from the sky (Figure 3.22).

The Alexander *monkey* position is similar. With a less wide stance, flex at ankles and knees and at the hip line, and incline forwards from the hips this time. Shoulders stay wide and lowered, abdominals firm, no kinks in the neck or back, and you extend headwards all along the spine. This is a strong and practical stance from which to use the

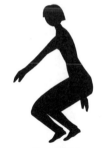

Figure 3.20

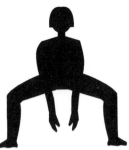

Figure 3.21

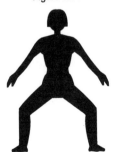

Figure 3.22

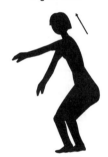

Figure 3.23

arms and can be shallow or quite deep (Figure 3.23).

Practising lowering the body in these several mechanically sound ways strengthens the legs and abdominals and re-educates the leg hinges. As they give us many useful reminders, the exercises insure against faulty use of the back. Try them at odd moments and use your own variations of them whenever you lower the body.

6: Fluid side-to-side whole body movement

The big bi-pedal movements used in the warming up sequence also belong in this section for the legs. Use them often, to stay flexible and to feel the connectedness and the flow of movement right through the body. The instructions are repeated here for ease of access and to give a little more detail.

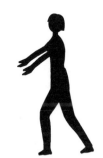

Figure 3.24

Stand with feet well apart. Share your weight evenly between the feet at first. Feel that your torso lifts out of a nice open pelvis.

Let both arms swing across the body to the right side, loosely. Turn the body towards the right and lift and turn the left heel as you turn so that both feet are following the direction of your arms (Figure 3.24).

Repeat freely and lightly from side to side.

Continue these swings, taking a wider stride as you gradually increase the range of movements. As you cross the centre line, begin to use the hinges of the legs to go deeper, and as you swing to either side reach higher and further round each time (Figure 3.25).

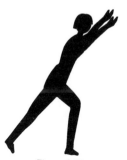

Figure 3.25

Increase the range until you are reaching as high and turning round as far as you can. Turn the head, as if to look up at the moon or the sky high behind you. Between these high reaches sink as low as your three leg hinges and released buttocks will take you (Figure 3.26).

Keep all movements soft, and feel the flow right through the body from feet to fingertips.

Finally, break out of the rhythm of this exercise

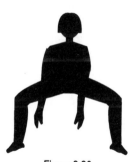

Figure 3.26

and move around the room with the same flow. Imagine placing things on high shelves and into low cupboards, and reaching behind, forwards, under and all around you. Take your weight from one foot to the other very smoothly with a flow of movement through the whole body, the foot direction guided by the direction of your attention and arm movement. With a similar extension, pretend that you are first giving something generously, then receiving something appreciatively.

Everyday Applications

Use flowing movements like these when picking flowers, making beds, planing wood, ironing, cleaning your teeth, opening a door, or for any other actions where movements from side to side and up and down are involved.

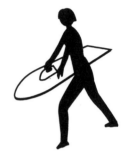

Figure 3.27

We are often recommended to rest one foot on a step when ironing. The danger with such *parking* is that the body may sink its weight into the hip joint. Ironing can become a pleasurably mobile and upright exercise if we resist slumping and take our weight openly and uprightly from one foot to the other. Keep the body relaxed, shoulders wide and lowered, and move smoothly with the action of ironing like the traditional wash-day song (Figure 3.27).

With feet and legs joining in with the arm movements the whole of you is involved. If some fore-and-aft movement is needed, use a small forward step and transfer your weight from front to back over the knee and ankle hinges, as in the ankle weighting exercises (Figure 3.28). Then change to side-to-side movements again, feet apart and knees directed out.

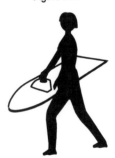

Figure 3.28

In some warmer countries women still wash their linen in a river or public wash place, singing as they work. This is even more of a whole-person activity. And it becomes a whole-group activity, too, strengthening connectedness in the community as an extra bonus.

Singing helps to free body movement and mind and spirit, too. It could also bring us much extra pleasure and right brain cooperation if we would use it more. I recommend singing or listening to music, or both, while *dashing along with the smoothing iron*.

EXERCISE SECTION 4

Hip Joints, Pelvis and Mid-back Flexibility

The Exercises

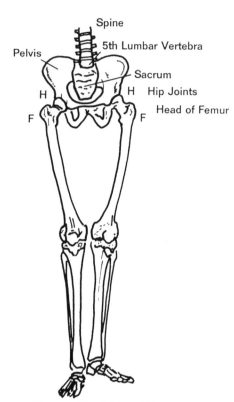

Spine

5th Lumbar Vertebra

Pelvis

Sacrum

H   H   Hip Joints

F   F   Head of Femur

Figure 4.1. The Pelvis as bridge

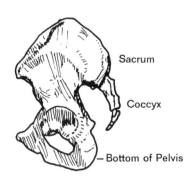

Sacrum

Coccyx

Bottom of Pelvis

Figure 4.2. Simplified drawing of Pelvis

Introduction

The pelvis bridges the legs and carries the weight of the spine and all the upper body above the arch it makes. Much of our movement depends on a smooth transfer of action through the hip joints and mid-back and it makes a big positive difference if we maintain flexibility here. Walking could never happen if our legs were rigid and hips fixed, and although it looks precarious, the engineering, well used, is remarkably efficient.

This pelvic arch from hip to hip is basically quite narrow, as the hip joints are deeply inset (Figure 4.1). The angled neck of the femur (F, F), gives the appearance of a wider base to the arch we stand on, but the pivots themselves are not wide apart. There would be extra problems in loading a wider arch. We can imagine the pressure of the weight of the torso and upper body straining the hip joints outwards if they were more widely set.

Our sitting span is even narrower, bridging the smaller gap between the tuberosities of the ischia or *sitting bones* (S, S), the strong bottom edges of the pelvis (Figure 4.2). The sacrum is the keystone for both arches.

It pays to get to know our joints, and this exercise programme is designed to help us to do this. If we have a faulty picture of where the hip or sitting bones are, we are less likely to use them well, but an accurate image encourages good use of the mechanics.

If we regularly sit rolled back on the curve of the sacrum and coccyx, we strain the lumbar vertebrae and the discs between them (Figure 4.3).

Regular exercise can help to keep our spinal flexibility, but we should also try to establish a good sitting posture as an every day positive contribution to mechanical good sense (Figure 4.4), and see Section 5b.

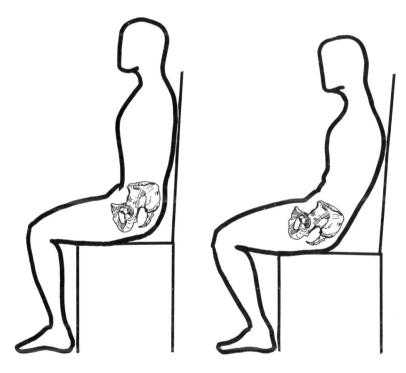

THIS WAY UP FOR THE PELVIS
WHEN SITTING

Figure 4.3

SLUMPING ON TO THE TAIL BONE
STRAINS THE VERTEBRAE AND
DISCS OF THE SPINE.

Figure 4.4

The Exercises

1: Exploring the hip joints

Standing

(a) Raise one knee, the thigh horizontal.
Circle this knee, one way and then the other, three
or four times (Figure 4.5). Repeat, drawing bigger
circles.
Repeat both movements for the other leg.

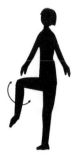

Figure 4.5

(b) *Paw the ground* with each leg in turn. Paw six
times towards you and then six times away (Figure 4.6).

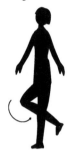

Figure 4.6

(c) Shake each leg in turn, loosely (Figure 4.7).

Lying

The first lying down movements repeat (a) and
(b) of the standing sequence, but now, unweighted, the hip is free to make bigger movements.

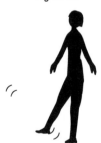

Figure 4.7

(a) Raise your right knee towards the ceiling, and
draw four or five small circles with it, first one
way and then the other. Then draw four or five
larger circles, again each way in turn (Figure 4.8).
These movements, as well as exercising and lu-
bricating the joint, help to give us a feeling for the
location of the hip joints so we become more
aware of them as we use them.

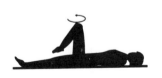

Figure 4.8

Next explore the whole range of movement available at the hip joint. Let the knee extend and flex and cross the body or reach out as you take it wherever it can go. Let your back roll a little as the hip explores its full range (Figure 4.9).

Rest the right leg and repeat both the small and large circles and all the larger movements for the left leg.

(b) Make pawing movements, six forwards and six back, for each leg in turn (Figure 4.10). Rest both legs.

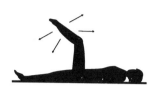

Figure 4.9

(c) Slide the right foot towards you with the knee out, sliding along the floor to your right side.

Raise the knee, leaving the foot on the mat, then slide the foot down beside the straight left leg (Figures 4.11 and 12).

Repeat this *knee out, knee up, leg slide* five times, and then repeat for the left leg.

Again, the exercise mobilises the joint, but it also lets the leg fall into its natural line of movement. After familiarising yourself with the action, repeat slowly, adding breath awareness, for five more complete cycles.

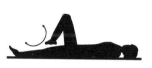

Figure 4.10

(d) Breathe in as you turn the knee out. Breathe in further as you bring it up. Lift the foot up this time and draw it as close to the buttocks as possible.

Breathe out as you lower the foot and slide it down and extend the heel away for fullest stretch of leg length.

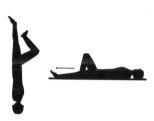

Figure 4.11

This leg slide with breathing is a good alignment exercise. As a bonus, it also extends awareness of the muscular support that the lower abdominals give to the breath, right down to the groin as the last traces of breath are expelled.

The exercise can also be done like a back stroke swimming movement, both legs drawing out together, lifting together and pushing down together. Start with two cycles and build up to five or more as the muscles strengthen.

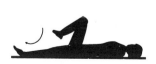

Figure 4.12

(e) Rock each leg in turn, loosely, all the way from the ankle to the hip socket (Figure 4.13).

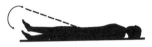

Figure 4.13

(f) Lift both knees, hold one in each hand, and stir them around. Use clockwise and anti-clockwise circles and figures of eight as well. Let the hips roll a little with all of these movements (Figure 4.14).

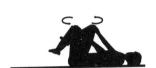

Figure 4.14

(g) Circle, kick and wave both legs together, unheld, in all directions (Figure 4.15).

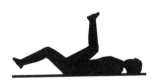

Figure 4.15

(h) With knees up, feet on the floor, roll the hips to one side. Let the head roll, too, and extend the top leg to kick loosely forwards across the body. Flex the knee again and roll back. Roll across to the other side and kick the other way. Keep the kicking leg quite close to the floor (Figure 4.16). Repeat four times.

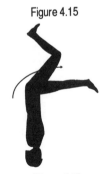

Figure 4.16

2: Hips, thighs and pelvis

These exercises are also valuable for releasing muscles of the outer thigh. Variation (ii) goes further still, giving a good stretch right across the body. Both should be done slowly to allow muscles to release.

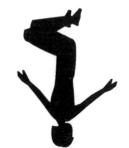

(i) A nice basic hip roll to do often. Lie with the knees up.

Roll your hips right over to the left (Figure 4.17).

Figure 4.17

Stay for a few seconds, to release the outer thigh muscles then return to the upright position. Relax again then roll to the right. Repeat the two rolls.

(ii) This extended variation gives a more comprehensive stretch but becomes quite easy with practice. Don't overstretch, but allow a gradual improvement each time you work with it.

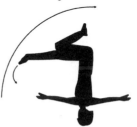

Lie with knees up, arms out to the sides.

Roll the hips to your left and let the head roll, too. Roll until your legs reach the floor. Your right shoulder will lift, as well as the hip to make this

Figure 4.18

big rotation possible, but fingertips should be able to stay on the floor (Figure 4.18).

Extend the upper leg slowly, relaxing in the hip joint and lengthening along the outer leg. At first the foot may not reach the floor. If you roll the hip a little further it should just touch. In this big extension right across the body you will also feel a widening stretch in the upper chest and shoulder.

Next, *walk* this foot up, chorus girl style, along the floor, with four little tapping steps towards the extended left hand. Quite a stretch!

Walk it back four steps towards the flexed left leg, and then raise and lower it four times.

During the toe tapping and leg raising, face towards the foot even though you cannot see it all the time.

Walk it down four or more little steps until in line with the body. Roll back and rest for a few moments with the left knee out to the side, the right leg extended (Figure 4.19). Enjoy the open stretch. Raise the knees, rest for a few moments, then repeat for the other side and again for both sides.

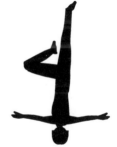

Figure 4.19

In the upper body work, there is a similar roll for the shoulders and neck. Sometimes take that exercise immediately after this one when both are familiar. Again, let your eyes follow the movement. There is a nice sense of connectedness in our body movements when the eyes join in. Staring takes away some of our awareness.

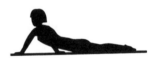

Figure 4.20

3: Exploring mid-back movement

(i) Lying on the stomach:

(a) With hands beside shoulders, push to arch the back and lengthen the whole front of the torso, pushing the chin forward and up (Figure 4.20). Hold for 10 counts.

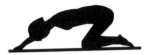

Figure 4.21

Feel the flexing in the mid-back as the front lengthens upwards. Return to the resting position.

(b) Lift head and shoulders, press on the hands to lift up and tuck back as in Figure 4.21. Use fingertips to push you further back until buttocks are back over the heels. Head relaxes down, elbows resting beside it.

Relax the elbows, let the spine lengthen, and stay relaxed for three full breaths or longer (Figure 4.22).

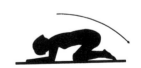

Figure 4.22

Repeat (a) and (b) then relax.

(ii) Kneeling, with light cushioning for the knees:

(a) Sit back on the heels, then lift up on to the knees, curl forwards and let the head fall to the mat, hands resting below the shoulders (Figure 4.23).

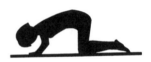

Push off with the hands, raise arms high and wide and gently open and lengthen your whole front, all the way from the knees to the chin and arch the back. The upper chest, especially, will widen right across to the shoulders and extending arms. Break

Figure 4.23

up the symmetry of this backward stretch by using a little side-to-side and rotational movement, the arms reaching back alternately as you gradually increase the stretch (Figure 4.24).

Return to the curled down position and repeat the arching back and curling down several times, slowly and smoothly.

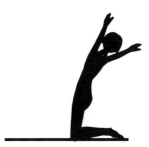

Figure 4.24

(b) Kneel on all fours with fists for support, knees apart, elbows bent slightly to flatten the back. Shoulders are wide and the spine long. Lift both feet and swing them from side to side, like wagging the tail, your head moving slightly, oppositely to the tail, six to eight times each way (Figure 4.25).

Vary the spinal twist. Turn head and tail together, to the same side, looking back under the arms, and twist from side to side.

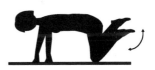

Figure 4.25

(iii) Standing:

(a) Take a long step forward on the right foot. Bend the front knee and move forward over it. Use hands on the knee to steady your balance. Press back with the back heel (Figure 4.26). The stretch is felt in the muscles of the left thigh. Don't over-stretch. Raise both arms loosely above the head, sink a little lower, and hold for a few seconds (Figure 4.27) Repeat for the other leg.

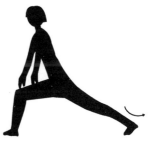

Figure 4.26

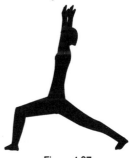

Figure 4.27

(b) Step forwards on the right again, but now place hands on hips and rotate the body to face left, opening out both pelvis and upper body. Bend the right knee, the torso staying upright. Hold for a few seconds in your deepest most open stretch (Figure 4.28).

Reverse the position and repeat.

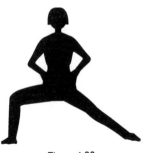

Figure 4.28

The Mid-Back and Posture – Everyday Reminders

The least stressful standing posture is a vertically resting one, with the main weights well aligned and the mid-back and abdominals long, strong and flexibly supportive. There are such obvious mechanical advantages in this that it is a pity not to use it. In fact, *posture* may be too static a word for this practical upright balance. There are no fixed relationships between the joints and muscles to be rigidly adhered to and there are personal differences between us too. The last thing we should do is to tighten the whole uprightness into ram-rod stiffness.

For a first level of postural upgrading, use a mirror to notice – non-judgmentally – if you habitually lean forwards or backwards, or twist or bend sideways, from the ankles, waist, hips or the mid or upper back. If leaning or rotating has become a habit it is a good idea to start to wonder why. Let the mind join in! Become observant of yourself and others.

Very often it is a social or psychological condition that leads our uprightness astray. We may react, or perhaps used to react in the past to some situations or people in certain ways, and have become stuck with the habit of doing that. It could well be that we no longer need to do it, and a few moments of enquiry can help to release it. If brave, ask someone else what they see in your ordinary standing position.

Psychology and Posture

It is a useful generalisation to think of a forward bowing lean as a slightly submissive posture, and a backward lean as somewhat defensive or perhaps a bluff of strength if the chest is thrown out too. These may not be the only reasons, and we do not make these variations consciously, but having adopted them unconsciously they can become annoyingly habitual.

Any lean however slight will need its own compensation in the tilt of the head, simply to allow us to look straight ahead rather than to the floor or the sky. So either position can lead to some shortening of neck and back or front and to increasing tension and fatigue, too.

As we don't actually need to be submissive or defensive, but best meet our fellow human beings straightforwardly, and especially as the balanced posture introduces no strain, the upright stance is more satisfactory all round. It looks better, too, and invites trust and confidence.

We can slowly recover a natural balance if we keep a good mental vision of it and think about our mechanical uprightness and our social ease together sometimes. Undoing bends and twists and opening out any inward shrinking compression can only bring a new physical health and a new directness to all our relationships.

Use the Level Head exercise from the warm-ups by a mirror for a postural reminder.

Making Changes

If you know you have an alignment habit to correct, even a small one, let the changes happen slowly. A lifetime of habit may lie behind our personal patterns and it takes time to shift them up in our awareness.

It can take courage, too, even to be willing to make positive changes. A sudden alteration can make us feel insecure and awkward. Even if a mirror shows that we are more upright after exercising, we may feel we are leaning in the opposite direction if we make a sudden change. I have seen people make a very positive difference to their posture in a class, and then leave, already adopting a bowed head position as they go out of the door. But gradually the habit has relaxed, practice and increasing suppleness have made way for changes, and lasting improvement has come.

This persistence of a habit is so usual that we must accept it graciously, with all the compromises that acceptance will involve. We are not looking for instant perfection, only for optimising the way our bodies minds and spirits can work together. Frustration and impatience only force further tensions and restraints, and manufacture bad chemistry, too. Be positively glad to shift quite slowly towards a more positive alignment and a more general level of fitness.

In brief, if we want to change a habit, of misalignment or anything else, it is easiest if:

❐ We are not self critical, but really want to make a positive change

❐ We are willing to do something active and positive about it and step up our effort in the matter

❐ We are not critical of others we see, either, but just wonder how their kinks came about and use their example only positively, to help us.

At a spiritual level, a sense of the equality of worth and the okayness of all other human beings is invaluable in freeing us for positive changes in ourselves. Look again at: "I am wrong!", "You are wrong!", "He or she or they are wrong!". These and all negative judgements introduce subtle tightnesses into bodies, minds and spirits.

Spiritual suppleness and *uprightness* only need awareness that they are available. They can be re-established just by switching over to them! When we make only enquiring and sympathetic observation of others and keep that *positive regard* alive for our fellow human beings, that plusness of spirit filters through to reinforce our physical integrity and fitness. It seems to be one of nature's lessons to us, certainly to me: that which we criticise in others often enters our own lives in quite disruptive ways. Either we attract and exhibit the same fault we criticised or, perhaps, we had that one already, and simply would not accept it in ourselves.

Forget about perfection, for there is no such thing in ourselves or others. But keep an eye on the general principles, bodily, mentally and spiritually, that work best, and in a good direction, for all of us. Our spine and posture benefit from any simple appreciation of the fact that uprightness, length, openness and suppleness are all natural to our species, lovely to see in others, and can be maintained by kindly observation and thoughtful exercise.

Backbone and Gender

An upright, mobile and alive posture is a statement of inner strength, yet we are sometimes quite afraid to be strong! Strength does not have to mean being domineering. It is part of our ability to give support to others and to make decisions and act independently or cooperatively in a very challenging world.

Men and women often differ in their deep seated attitudes to strength, because of our different biological history and traditional cultural roles. Men display their strength more, and more often use it competitively. In the past they were actively ready to protect the more vulnerable and dependent female.

Some women today are keen to emphasise strength and power and show men that they are not dependent or inferior. Some others, even in today's fast changing culture, often fear that an appearance of strength is either unwomanly or will be perceived as an actual threat to other men or women. Others are just naturally inclined to seek cooperation and do not want to seem threatening.

These deep-seated gender differences and our more recent adaptations creep into our actions and muscle tone subconsciously. But genes and culture need not dictate destiny! With increasing body awareness we can make slow changes and remake some of our own attitudes. With imagination and thought, we can find a wholesomely appropriate strength. Men can choose to use their backbone strengths in more generally supportive ways today, and women who may have been very compliant can learn to use theirs more assertively sometimes.

All the exercises of this section can be used to restore our inner strength as well as our suppleness to a level that is natural and appropriate for us and good to work with.

Rigidity and weakness are the two extremes for the body/mind and they both restrict us. At our core or backbone, human beings of both sexes, need both flexibility and strength. We need the ability to stand firmly on our own feet and power our own convictions, but also the good sense to cooperate or even to give way when that will bring a greater good.

EXERCISE SECTION 5A

Mid-torso Work, the Abdominal Group

The Exercises

Introduction

The exercises of this section are designed to maintain the length and tone of the muscles of the abdomen, and to increase awareness of their use.

The muscles here, act like a layered sheath, providing strength and flexibility. They share in the work of locomotion and breathing, contain the inner organs and assist in stabilising the spine.

The transverse muscles are the deepest of the abdominals, running from the spine round to the centre front. The internal oblique muscles wrap diagonally over the transverse ones. The external obliques cover the internal obliques, and, lastly, the long straight pair of rectus abdominis muscles extend upwards from the pubic bone, on either side of the mid-line, fanning out to attach to the ribs (see page 44).

A possible risk in exercising the abdominals is that of disproportionately exaggerating the strength of the rectus abdominis. This muscle is used to draw the ribs towards the pelvis, and if we exercise it while shortening our front length, the whole torso may tend to shorten, and this will bring many problems.

It is also practical to consider that if the rib cage itself is tight it may tighten the shoulders and narrow them. In this case the abdomen will probably protrude more than it need. So these exercises should be backed up by some to loosen up the ribs and free the shoulders to widen naturally.

The Exercises

These follow easily from the previous section, or they can be done as a separate unit.

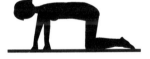

1: Kneeling – use a small cushion for the knees

(a) Take up an *all fours* position, knees a little apart, fists well ahead, supporting a long flat back, neck in line with the spine (Figure 5A.1). Fists are better than flat hands for support, as the wrist suffers less strain if used as shown.

Figure 5.A.1

Breathe in, arch up, pull in the abdominals and hold the pull for a count of six or more, while breathing out (Figure 5A.2). Relax. Repeat four times.

(b) Breathe in, arch up again, tighten the abdominals, and on the out breath, move your body weight forward between the arms, lengthening the long front muscles. Hold for a count of six, while ex-

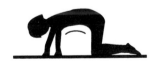

Figure 5.A.2

haling (Figure 5A.3). Relax back, then repeat four times slowly.

2: Lying

Do this group of four exercises every day if your abdominals need a tonic. The variety of positions is important. Their order is less important. None of them scrunches the abdominals into shortened toning.

(i) Start with the knees out, the soles of the feet touching.

Figure 5.A.3

Lengthen the torso and tuck shoulder blades under. Place both hands behind the neck, elbows out, the hands not linked but overlapping.

Breathe in, using the action of inhaling to lift the sternum and increase the front length slightly. Start to breathe out and start to tighten the abdomen, for the first three counts of exhaling.

As you continue to exhale and continue to tighten, lift just the shoulders and head. Hold for five counts, still releasing the breath (Figure 5A.4). Relax. Repeat four times.

Figure 5.A.4

(ii) Lie with right leg extended. Place the left heel on the mat beside the right mid-calf, with the left knee up. Support your head as before. (Figure 5A.5).

Use the same lengthened torso and same three-stage breathing cycle as before but this time add leg-raising to the work the muscles have to do.

Breathe in, lengthening the front. Start to breathe out and to tighten the front muscles, for three counts. Continuing to tighten and exhale, raise the head and shoulders as before and also raise the right leg, well extended, to about 6 to 12 inches from the floor. Look towards the foot. Hold for five counts (Figure 5A.6). Lower the leg slowly, relax and repeat the whole movement four times.

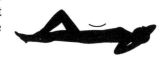

Figure 5.A.5

Repeat for the left leg.

The foot on the mat should exert a small heel pressure downwards as you extend the raised leg.

Figure 5.A.6

This helps it to lengthen all the way out from the hip, and it also assists the abdominal muscle support.

(iii) Lie with both legs extended at first. With the same breathing cycle and slight downward pressure from the left heel, raise the head and your extended right leg as before and hold for five counts (Figure 5A.7). Repeat for the left leg.

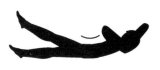

Figure 5.A.7

Alternate the leg raising this time and complete five cycles. Don't hurry! Each movement needs to start with the torso lightly lengthened for the inhalation, and the exhalation starts before you raise your head and the leg, each time.

(iv) Lie with both legs extended, head supported as before. This time, lengthen, breathe in, start to breathe out and tighten the abdominals, then simply raise head and shoulders with no leg raising, and look towards your upturned feet. Hold for a count of five, relax. Repeat this cycle four times, or more.

Repetitions

The number of repetitions for this group of abdominal exercises can be increased, little by little, if you want to make real progress with them, to 10, 20, or more. Or repeat them later in the day. Don't hurry them, even for a longer sequence. Always take time to work consciously with the breath and muscles, and to appreciate the good work you are doing.

If you do a lot of repetitions, keep your arms by your sides and make a definite break to walk around for about half a minute between the groups. In a more general workout programme the smaller number suggested here will keep you in trim and can be done with just a short pause between the exercises.

(v) Arm and leg raise and lower – lying on the mat.

Only do this exercise when you are comfortable with the earlier ones, and feel the need of a bigger challenge. Then only build up to five repetitions quite slowly. It is a stronger exercise, and builds muscle strength, but not one to do if you are exercising newly. By raising the legs separately from a raised knee start, the abdominals are not over-strained, and the main work is done as you lower the four limbs approximately together.

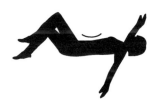

Lie with knees raised, feet apart, arms widely spread (Figure 5A.8).

Figure 5.A.8

Start with an in-breath, lengthening as before. As you start to breathe out begin to tighten the abdominals, for three counts.

Still exhaling, lift your head and shoulders well up first, then one limb after another, in any order, as shown (Figure 5A.9).

Hold the extended starfish position momentarily, then lower arms and legs and head together gently as the breath is fully released.

Rest for a few moments. Raise the knees to the starting position, and repeat. At first, one repetition is enough, Build up to a longer hold time first, and then to five repetitions, over some time.

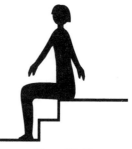

Figure 5.A.9

3: On an exercise bench or at the top of a stairway

Again, this exercise and its variations are strong ones and should only be done after some regular practice with the first, easier ones.

Sit first, with the sitting bones right on the edge of the bench or top of stairs (Figure 5A.10). Rest your feet, hip width apart, on the floor or on the second step down, directing the knees slightly outwards.

Figure 5.A.10

Lie back, readjust to bring your sitting bones even closer to the edge. Lengthen the back. Tuck shoulder blades under. Feel the slight natural arching between sacrum and shoulders (Figure 5A.11).

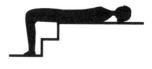

Breathe in, lightly extending the front. Start to exhale, tightening the abdominals. Three counts. Hold for six more counts, breathing out. Relax. Repeat six times.

Figure 5.A.11

Variation 1

Repeat the above exercise with arms extended along the floor or bench behind your head.

Variation 2

Supporting your head with overlapped hands, lift head and shoulders during the six counts of maximum work for the abdominals (Figure 5A.12). Repeat three times.

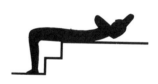

4: Oblique muscles sequence – lying

Figure 5.A.12

This basic exercise and its extended version is for everybody! Easy but very effective. Breathe normally.

(i) Lie with knees up, feet together, arms wrapped above the head, torso long. Shoulders stay on the mat.

Let the knees roll slowly from one side to the other. The left hip lifts from the mat as you roll to the right, and vice versa. Relax as you lower the knees to the floor, but use the abdominal muscles as you lift the knees up, feeling the oblique stretch. Repeat for five complete cycles (Figure 5A.13).

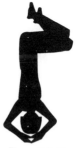

Figure 5.A.13

(ii) This is simply a nice extended version of (i). Allow more time for it. We progressively change the starting position to increase the range of muscles exercised, and by rolling the head oppositely, give the muscles between the ribs a little stretch as well.

(a) Start with the knees raised as in (i), but at a very shallow angle this time. As in (i), roll the legs slowly to one side, pause and relax there, lift them to the centre, then roll them to the opposite side, pause, and lift back to the centre again, eight times (four cycles). Keep the neck free. Let your head roll oppositely to the roll of the hips. End with knees raised, and relax.

(b) Draw feet a few inches closer to the buttocks, then step them just a little wider apart, and repeat the movements. Make sure to relax in the hip joint, and encourage the upper leg to relax as it follows the lower one to the floor.

Do four cycles, ending with the knees up. Relax.

(c) Draw the feet a little closer still and step them a little further apart. Repeat as above.

(d) Draw the feet as close as possible to the buttocks and step them as far apart as they will go. Relax, then roll the knees slowly from side to side. At the lowest point, feet roll right on to their sides while the upper leg relaxes towards the floor. During the pause, try to let go of any tension and enjoy the stretch. Complete four cycles. Relax.

As this exercise becomes familiar you will enjoy the increased flexibility it brings to hips and waist, and rib cage too. Build up to 10 or more repetitions at each position, to work these muscles well.

5: Seated exercises

(i) The Aware Pull-In

Sit on a firm chair, balancing the spine vertically above the sitting bones. Lengthen and widen both back and front, lifting the lower torso out of the hips, and the upper torso out of the waist. Don't try too hard. Check that the back does not arch back or the neck tighten. The head should stay level, not arched back. Shoulders are wide and lowered, hands relaxed on your lap.

Now, with no preparatory in-breath, just exhale and pull in the lower abdominal muscles, drawing the abdominal wall towards the spine. Drop your shoulders. Release neck and shoulder tension. Hold for a few moments, then relax and pause. Lengthen up again as a natural in-breath returns, and wait for a partial easy outflow before starting the next pull. Repeat several times, slowly, with pauses.

This exercise can be done while driving, or at a desk or even a dinner table. In all of these situations it gives you a nice postural check, and at meal times it can act as a useful reminder not to overload the food processing department!

(ii) Reaching from a sitting position

Lengthening upwards, inhale, draw in the muscles of the abdomen as before, and then extend your torso forwards, hinging at the hips. Avoid neck tension by letting the head tip forwards as you lean (Figure 5A.14).

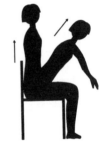

Explore the entire range of the reach of your arms in all directions, including under the chair. Feel your weight move from one sitting bone and buttock to the other as you reach from side to side.

For **shoe-tying:**

Use the long forward reach of this exercise, when fastening your shoes, before curving shoulders down. Lengthen towards one knee and then the

Figure 5A.14

other. The short cut of curling down from a slumped posture leads to compression in the abdomen and lower back. Try both ways and notice the difference (Figs 5A.15 and 16).

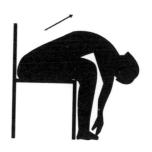

Figure 5A.15

6: Walking abdominal exercise

Walk in an easy relaxed upright way, just being yourself. Undo any tightness in seat muscles or thighs. Check for neck tension by resting the finger tips lightly along the back of the neck and release that tension. Avoid tilting or thrusting the head back or forwards. But it is not practical to try to be perfect! Once major neck tensions are avoided, relax and do the abdominal exercise quite slowly, just as you are.

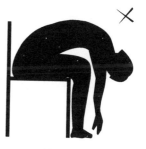

Figure 5A.16

Feel some vertical but not exaggerated or arched lift in your walk, and alternately contract and relax the abdomen below the navel while you walk. Take four slow steps with tightened abdominals as you breathe out, and four more with slack muscles as you breathe in. Imagine your in-breath filling the expanding lower abdomen and expanding the ribs to the sides and the back. The out-breath starts in the lower abdomen and closes the ribs. Do several cycles. Play with slowing or speeding your walk, and finally try to maintain just a little extra, non-exaggerated tone in the abdominals as an extra spinal support all the time, breathing naturally.

Benefits: When we deliberately lengthen and exercise the abdominal muscles it wakes them up for us. Exercising them in the condition of normal use shows us their range of ability in a way that the body remembers. Use them all regularly, the walking one on everyday walks, and the seated ones at your desk or at meal times. The more aware we become of them, the more these muscles will remember to play their full threefold part in containing the inner organs properly, supporting the balance of the spine, and assisting our breathing, whether walking, standing or sitting.

EXERCISE SECTION 5B

Torso and Spine/Sitting and Stretching

Everyday Sitting

The practice of sitting is comparatively recent in the evolutionary time scale. It is a specifically human posture. Most of the human race has now changed away from the deep squatting way of resting. But chairs are often taken as an opportunity to slump, and slumping creates havoc with backs and insides. The human spine could benefit from a little more squatting.

To get away from the slump into the pelvis that sitting so often becomes, we should aim to use our extension between sitting bones and the sky, even while firmly seated. The combination of becoming aware, getting the conditions right and then using a little positive vision and choice in the matter, can work this transformation for us. There is a lot of detail to think about before we exercise specifically for this section.

We have seen that we cannot help the anti-gravity muscles directly. We need to be aware of, sympathetic to and not interfering with them. They work well and beautifully if we let them operate naturally.

Forcing the body, trying too hard, and contracting, shrinking or collapsing, all tighten muscles, and we know that prolonged tightening inevitably damages them. Once again, it takes time to make improvements if we have a long-standing habit to change, and we may have to accept some compromise along the way. It really does pay us good dividends when we enjoy each small improvement for itself, whenever it comes.

Think about the extra strain involved when you ask those sensitively balanced anti-gravity muscles to carry the weight of your head and arms right outside the line of best mechanical strength. Notice the way weight then gets transferred to muscles and ligaments that need not be strained.

Ligaments are meant to be last ditch supports! They are there, for example, to hold your head on when the muscles that should be doing that job are excessively stretched or damaged, as in a sudden accident. If we ask them to support the head far out of line all the time, they will stiffen as do other connective tissues, and the muscles designed for the task give up. All the connective tissues between and around misused or neglected muscles gradually harden and lose their elasticity. And then the trouble begins.

Positive images and cheerful attitudes encourage and help us towards positive change. Rest lightly upwards when you remember, and then remember more often!

The following practical guidelines are a useful consciousness exercise for sitting. They do not define an exact posture because we all start from different places. Once in a while, take time to follow them right through and explore each one. The words I have stressed below involve some mental work.

(i) *Be aware* of the sitting base and your upright spine above it. Choose a level or slightly forward sloping and firm seat, high enough to let your knees rest a little lower than the hips, feet flat and relaxed on the floor. Sit on the edge of the chair for this exploration.

Separate the legs a little and direct feet and knees slightly outwards. Let go of any thigh tension. Imagine the upper body is *standing* vertically and unskewed above the sitting bones and the pelvic arch.

Make sure you are neither arching the back nor trying to roll back on the coccyx. Remember, too, that although the spine provides both flexibility and a firm line of support, when sitting we need the support strength more than the flexibility. Minimise that natural curve of the back without forcing your straightness. See illustrations of Section 4.

The bottom edges of the ischial tuberosities have a useful curve. If we balance above that support and use the abdominals, too, we can achieve a strong vertical line. Tuck one hand under your buttocks to locate one of these bones and you can feel it move back as you lean forwards and forwards as you lean back. Stay with it at the lowest point.

(ii) *Think about* the anti-gravity system operating all the way up the spine to the muscles that adjust the balance of the head, and *trust* it to work well. *Imagine* and *appreciate* it doing a good job for you.

(iii) *Check* all through the body for any holding tension anywhere. Include feet, legs, buttocks, shoulders, neck, jaw, tongue, hands and eyes, but use just a little extra abdominal tone to give your spine light support.

(iv) *Intend* your direction to be upwards and widthways, lengthening up and widening across pelvis, lower and mid back, upper chest and shoulders.

If thinking about upward movement makes your back arch and your head tip back, lower the chin lightly. If the lowered chin brings your eyes downwards, adjust them to the new position last. If your eyebrows frown down, lift and widen them, brighten your eyes and cheer up! Check for neck tension by placing soft fingertips along the neck vertebrae, and release it if tight.

Feel the back of the neck lengthening up, as if all the way from between the shoulder blades, while the balanced yoke of the shoulders relaxes out and down. Feel proud and very much alive!

(v) *Introduce small movements* from time to time, to avoid rigidity. Make some tiny movements to nod and turn your head high on its top vertebrae to keep the neck free and the head level.

To summarise the five awareness steps, they are: awareness, in turn, of sitting bones, anti-gravity system, tension release, upward and outwardness and remembering to make small movements to avoid rigidity.

F.M Alexander's basic directions to his pupils were to "free the neck and lengthen and widen the back". When backs have adopted a forward curve they already exceed the front in length. So it helps to think of lengthening and widening the whole front and sides of the torso together, to equalise front and back as well as bringing the back upright.

If the back has a tendency to arch back, which shortens it, it will be the front that needs restraint as you let the back find its proper length. Neither back nor front should lengthen or widen at the other's expense.

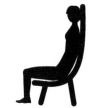

Figure 5.B.1

Try placing one spread hand on your upper chest and the other on the upper back and play with expanding one of those areas, then the other and then both together. The only scope for expansion if they are not to restrict each other, is in lengthening up together and widening out towards shoulder caps together.

Use these notes mostly as mental rather than physical exercises. There is not much *doing* here, but quite a lot of attention to give. Return to them often as part of a process of exploring and slowly improving your own best sitting posture.

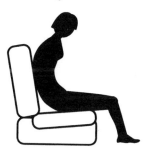

Figure 5.B.2

Adapting the Chair

Figures 5B.1 and 5B.2 show exaggerated versions of the sort of seats that present our backs with awkward conditions, especially in cars or aeroplanes. This is not the designer's intention, of course. He or she thinks we will be luxuriously happy with a hollowed out seat or a sloping back. In fact, we rest much better in nicely aligned extension whether sitting, standing or lying.

Figure 5B.3 shows how cushions can be used to fill up a too hollow or sloped seat or back.

Figure 5B.4 shows the use of a wedge of firm foam to give a slight forward tilt for dining or working. Figure 5B.5 shows how lengthening the back legs of a chair can do the same job.

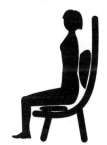

Figure 5.B.3

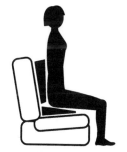

Figure 5.B.4

As a slumped sitting position creates problems for arm use as well as for backs, necks and all the inner organs, remember when using the arms, whether for holding a newspaper, driving a car, typing, playing the piano or chopping up carrots, to lift and widen the upper chest so the shoulder line rests across the upright spine. Your arms will then be free and wonderfully light in use. Check sometimes with one hand reaching to your spine, that you do not kink or *break* the line of the mid-back as part of the movement of arm lifting. Over-arching the back, as well as slumping forward with a rounded back, will strain it (Figures 5B.6 and 7).

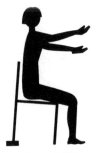

Figure 5.B.5

Can I Never Slump?

There are times when we only want to enjoy total laziness! If you cannot choose a horizontal rest – it is possible to watch the television lying down – try this halfway position in a chair with a high back. It allows you to rest back without too much compression or collapse.

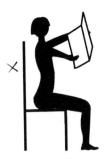

Figure 5.B.6

Adopt a really collapsed slump first, the front all folded down and shoulders rounded in. Then extend upwards, widen the upper body, and lean forwards from hip level, fully lengthened, abdominals helping the spine.

Then carry that length up again and back until your wide shoulders touch the back of the chair. Now with shoulder blades back and upper chest wide let your mid section release into a partial slump. This halfway measure still gives the insides some length and space.

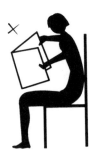

Figure 5.B.7

Torso Stretches, Front Back and Sides

1: Standing side stretches

(a) With feet a little apart, lift the right arm loosely, vertically up, palm in. Move your shoulder slightly back on that side, the inner arm beside the ear. Take your weight back a little and pull in the tummy. To align the spine, arch the back first and then unarch it, resting the head slightly forwards. If you bring the left hand up to the right shoulder blade or mid-back it can detect any over-arching and release it. Feel a gentle stretch from the foot below, all the way up your side (Figure 5B.8).

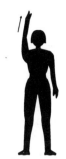

Figure 5.B.8

Tilt to your left increasing the stretch along the right side. Stay grounded in both feet, with no rotation of the torso. Take two full breaths in this stretched position to expand the right rib cage gently (Figure 5B.9). Return slowly to upright, lower the right arm and repeat for the left side.

(b) Stand with the legs wider astride, weight a little back. Smooth the lower back lightly down to straighten it, lowering the tail bones without tucking the pelvis hard under. Feel tall, and nice and wide across pelvis, midriff, upper chest and shoulders, both at the back and front.

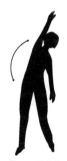

Figure 5.B.9

Turn your head to the right and lift the right hand, palm up, to shoulder level. Look towards it, and as you slowly tilt your torso to the left, lift the right hand and watch it all the way over. Stay grounded in both feet and avoid rotating at the waist. Imagine you are held between two big panes of glass (Figure 5B.10).

Extend the fingers, take two full expanding breaths, and then return slowly. Watch your extended hand return back to shoulder level then lower it to your side.

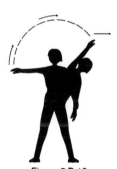

Figure 5.B.10

Repeat to the other side, and then repeat both ways.

2: Standing front stretch

Stand facing a wall, feet about 1ft from it, both hands resting on the wall at chest level. Lean from the ankles taking the pelvis towards the wall.

Keeping the left leg straight, step the right foot nearer to the wall. Transfer most of your weight to the right foot.

Now slide the right hand up the wall, reach high and then lean the open chest back away from the wall.

The right side stretches up, arching back in one long curve from ankles to fingertips. Left heel will lift to give you extra length. Look up, keeping the neck long, not hunched, and hold the stretch for a few seconds (Figure 5B.11). Lower the arm, reverse the foot positions, and repeat for left front stretch.

Repeat both stretches.

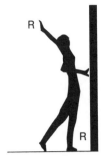

Figure 5.B.11

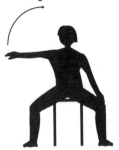

Figure 5.B.12

3: Seated side/back stretch

Sit uprightly on a firm seat, feet wide apart, spine balanced vertically above the sitting bones, left hand resting on the thigh, just above the left knee (Figure 5B.12). Turn to the right, open the upper body and circle your right hand and arm back, far round to your right (Fig 5B.13). Head follows the movement.

Complete a big circle, bringing the hand high up, then over and across you and diagonally forward.

Lean and lengthen forward to the left as the right arm stretches along this diagonal in a line well outside the left hand and knee (Figure 5B.14).

Hold the stretch for 10 counts. Repeat on the other side. Then repeat for each side once more.

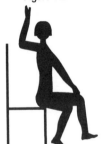

Figure 5.B.13

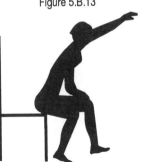

Figure 5.B.14

4: Seated stretch for the lower back

Sit with feet apart, hands on knees.

(i) Breathe in and lengthen up.

(ii) As you breathe out, lean and turn and extend your torso forwards over the left knee until nearly horizontal (Figure 5B.15).

(iii) Breathe in again, letting the top part of the torso, neck and shoulders, curl down (Figure 5B.16).

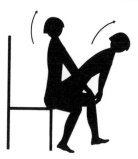

Figure 5.B.15

(iv) Reach hands to hold the toes of the left foot and, breathing out, lengthen forward, and pull on the front of the foot. You will feel the stretch in the lower back. Take two full breaths as you stretch.

Relax, return slowly to upright. Repeat once and then repeat to the right side. If you have differences in the mobility of the two sides, or cannot reach the toes first time, don't force this exercise. Think about releasing the lower back, appreciate even the slightest release, and be patient and confident that improvement will come with continued practice.

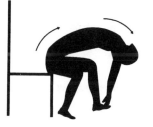

Figure 5.B.16

5: Seated stretch, lengthening up

Lift your hands out to your sides and over the head and rest the overlapping arms on top of the head. Maintain spine and neck length without arching either. The chin is slightly down (Figure 5B.17).

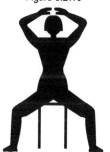

Figure 5.B.17

Now use an upward and side to side rocking lift to lengthen the middle torso. Pull in the abdominal muscles. Hold the central stretch for two full breaths (Figure 5B.18).

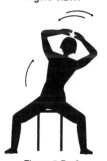

Figure 5.B.18

Lift the hands towards the ceiling again, turn the palms out, and then lower them, palms down, out and slowly down (Figure 5B.19).

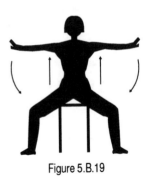

As the upward stretch may tend to hunch the neck into the shoulders, make a deliberate exercise on the way down of lengthening the back of both neck and upper back, keeping the face level and forwards.

Repeat the exercise and adopt it often, especially to interrupt long periods of desk work.

Figure 5.B.19

If you are tempted to kink or overarch the back for this exercise – which shortens the back – try it with one arm on the head and the other spread behind your back and shoulder to control the arching.

6: Back stretch with support

Use a hand rail, other fixture or the firm support of a partner who should use the strong foot position shown, one foot ahead of the other.

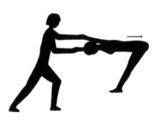

Stretch forwards from the hips with feet parallel and a little apart, holding on to the support firmly with extended arms (Figure 5B.20). Release the seat muscles to extend back, adjusting your distance from the support if necessary until you feel a good stretch all along the spine. Hold for 10 to 20 seconds. This is a wonderful stretch for a tired back.

Figure 5.B.20

Benefits and Everyday Applications

Whenever we stretch muscles a little further than usual, without strain, it reminds us that we do have that capacity and it helps to make our ordinary day-to-day use of them easier. Circulation is improved, oxygen supplies ensured, and waste chemicals will more easily be drained away.

Mechanically, all the midriff stretches make excellent antidote exercises to counteract the everyday risk of spinal compression. This happens so easily from prolonged sitting or from general inactivity. Mentally, just thinking about length and width is important.

You will enjoy regaining middle section length and flexibility. The exercises make a lot of positive difference to posture, lightness and our all-the-time ease of movement if we persist with them.

Fit these many stretches into little gaps in daily activities. No one will mind if you stretch in the car park after sitting in the driver or passenger seat for a long time. Add some big yawns and some general loosening up movements, too. You will be in a much better condition for walking, whether to the shops or over the hills and far away.

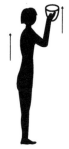

Use a coffee, tea or water break for another simple reminder of length while sitting or standing. Lengthen up first, then lift the cup or glass above your mouth as if to drink a toast. Avoid arching the back with this lifting movement. Pause momentarily, perhaps toast your own health while noticing this nice upward lift (Figure 5B.21).

Figure 5.B.21

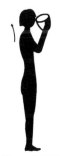

Then lower the cup very lightly to your lips with the slightest downward tilt of the chin (Figure 5B.22). Continue to lengthen up as you take your first sip and continue to drink. This is much

Figure 5.B.22

better than curling down to meet the cup and then kinking the back, and shortening the neck as you drink.

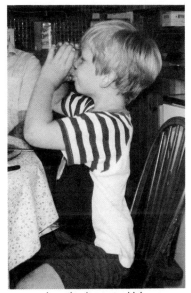

Lengthening up to drink

Introduction

This group starts with some use of weights for toning and strengthening the upper body and arms. It includes loosening up exercises for joints and stretching movements for muscles. It ends with some consciousness raising exercises for the hands.

The Upper Body and Posture

Many of our sporting activities such as running, and fast or long distance walking, are *leg sports*. These are excellent for building strength and stamina but can lead to an imbalance of muscle tone between upper and lower body if they are our sole exercise. Hamstrings and lower back and neck muscles can shorten and tighten, and then the posture may suffer. But we can help to avoid this imbalance by keeping the leg muscles loosened up and by making sure to exercise the upper body as well.

Non-competitive swimming is a good sport for posture, because of the way it involves upper and lower body together. We can adjust our personal sport and exercise programme to respect this important balance of fitness between upper and lower halves. I have introduced a vertical ladder at home for an alternative route upstairs. Climbing extends us well, and its use of arms and legs is a balanced one.

Body, Mind and Spirit Considerations

Holistic fitness involves physical, mental and spiritual coordination and co-operation continuously, all the time. Psychological, emotional and many other pressures often show up in bodily disfunction. Sexual anxiety can bring tensions to the lower torso, tightening the pelvic and leg muscles. Social and emotional stresses and fears can affect breathing and lead to upper body tensions with restrictions in the chest, jaw, hands, shoulders and neck. We can shrink physically from fears and anxieties. We can stoop unconsciously from feeling or even imagining ourselves to be unduly burdened. Quite small stresses can become the start of patterns of conditioning that become trapped in our muscles and may last a lifetime.

Among the stresses of spirit, I tend to include tight-fistedness or other meannesses of spirit in relation to others or even ourselves. I am sure we can exercise towards opening up this part of us into human generosity between people, as well as towards the joints, muscles and space-needing organs within. In this mechanistic world, even church leaders tread carefully or apologetically sometimes when they talk about spirits! It is the acknowledged *human spirit* that I speak of here, because we all know we have something about us that could accept that name. At times of crisis, illness, danger or death we may dare to talk of someone's spirit. While still alive and well we may also be able to nourish it.

These body/mind and spirit connections can work both ways. We know that bodily improvements often follow improved psychological health after counselling or other therapy, perhaps, religious conversion, just by switching to more positive attitudes, or even hearing some good news. If we become more accepting of and generous towards the child we were, the person we are now, other people in our life or the circumstances of our past and present life, we may shed some very deep muscle tensions. We may have watched a friend recover from a depression, for example, and noticed that posture, general movement and facial expressiveness all brighten and lighten as they start to feel better. We may have had or read about a transcendental experience and observed the physical radiance, if only in religious paintings, that comes with spiritual bliss.

It is not so obvious, perhaps, but it is also true, that healing can work the other way round too. By working from the bodily direction, upgrading suppleness, developing freer movement, fuller breathing and a more relaxed and balanced posture, people become better able to shed quite deep-seated psychological and emotional problems and become more open to the flow of spirit in the world.

Self awareness and acceptance, self confidence, and respect can all blossom, simply from the shedding of associated patterns of body tensions. Exercise, especially upper body exercise, works for us in all these areas.

Although psychological shifts can happen suddenly and dramatically sometimes with much emotional release, more usually the lightening up of minds and spirits is a gradually progressive process. We can wake up one morning and realise that an old anxiety has simply evaporated and life has taken on a rosier hue. In Tai Chi they speak of a bubble that rises to the surface and then disappears.

These upper body exercises especially need to honour the physical openness and length of the human torso and limbs with all the *plusness* you can make. Think all the time about lengthening and widening easily, up through the spine and across the open upper chest. Use the abdominal muscles to help to stabilise the spine. And have in mind the non-bodily bonuses: enhancing your ability to handle challenge, change and stress, building self esteem, improving the quality of your relationships and interactions with others, opening your whole life to a richer quality. How's that for positive motivation!

Don't Neglect the hands

Hands have special significance in all the shared higher human activities of nurturing and giving and receiving. When we *shake hands* we are making a link between ourselves and another human being. There is a spiritual dimension to these inter-human activities, a gap-crossing ability.

The nerve connections from the hands to the cortex are as complex and numerous as those of the highly developed senses of sight and hearing. Hands are very sensitive indeed. I have included hand exercises in this section, both to lighten our use of them and to make our everyday use of hands more conscious.

As well as gaining in dexterity and keeping arthritis at bay, when we free up joints and muscles of the hands we are freeing the spiritual member of our B/M/S team. Our human generosity, sensitivity and expressiveness are all being enlarged and opened as hands give up their tensions and become aware of their ability to be a part of our general extension in body, mind and spirit.

Hands have a leading role in our lives. While your head leads the body into action and floats your movement along, your hand can lead your arm. Send it lightly ahead, fingers first, when you reach for anything, from the alarm clock in the morning, opening up the curtains to welcome the day, caressing the steering wheel on the way to work, or reaching to the light switch for lights off at night.

The Exercises

1: With weights – for openness and muscle toning

Use the tins of beans, or weights of about 1 lb. Only increase these, to not more than 3 lb., if you feel strong or if the smaller ones come to feel too light.

(i) Stand uprightly but relaxed, feet apart. Hold the weights at chest level, hands wrapping softly round them, not grasping tightly (Figure 6.1).

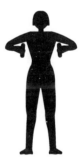

Figure 6.1

Reach to the side, extending one arm lightly, transferring your body weight that way as well, and letting the movement flow through the body. Look towards the extended hand (Figure 6.2).

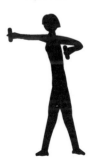

Figure 6.2

Next draw this weight in towards the chest and extend the other weight out to the other side, turning to watch the changeover and moving lightly in that direction (Figure 6.3).

Repeat for four or five cycles or more.

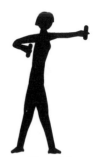

Figure 6.3

(ii) Hold the weight in the left hand in front of the body, and the other behind your back. Take a wider stance than before, transfer body weight over the left foot, bending the left knee (Figure 6.4).

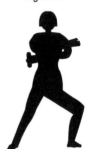

Figure 6.4

Now transfer your body weight to the right, ex-changing the position of the weights (Figure 6.5).

Repeat this exchange for four or five cycles.

Keep the movements wide and soft, and allow a slight rhythmic bounce at each changeover.

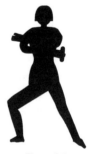

Figure 6.5

(iii) Under and overarm circling.

In a forward stride, left knee bent and in front, swing the weight in the right hand loosely for-wards across the body, then up and round and back in a full underarm circle. Your weight travels from the front foot to the back foot for support. Open the whole torso and shoulder area and follow the big movement right round with head and eyes (Figure 6.6).

Much of the momentum for the swing comes from

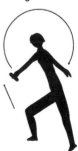

Figure 6.6

the springiness of the weighted foot on the floor. The front foot powers the underarm circle. The rear foot will take over when you reverse the direction. The whole body joins in with these big swings.

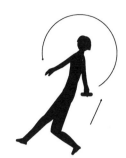

Repeat three times then change direction of the swing for four overarm circles, starting with your weight over the rear foot (Figure 6.7) As with overarm bowling, the rear foot is powering the action.

Figure 6.7

Repeat both under and over-arm circles with the left arm.

(iv) Lifting the weights.

(a) Hold the weight in the right hand at right shoulder level, the back unarched, then raise and lower it six times (Figure 6.8). Don't hurry or jerk the movements. Repeat the exercise for the left arm.

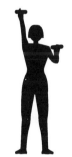

Figure 6.8

(b) Stand evenly weighted, pelvis vertical, back not arched. Lift the right elbow above your right shoulder, lowering the weight to behind the shoulder (Figure 6.9).

Raise the weight high up from this position and lower it again, six times altogether, and then repeat for the left arm. Keep the movements non-jerky but strong.

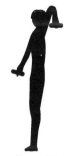

Figure 6.9

2: Shoulder shrugs, seated

(i) Circling one shoulder.

Sit uprightly, your weight carried above the sitting bones. Direct the right shoulder in and forwards, then lift it, rotate it slowly back and press it well down at the back. Don't lock the neck. Let the head turn a little and the upper body open out with the shoulder movement.

Complete four big circles then repeat for the other shoulder. Finally repeat the movements in the reverse direction, circling each shoulder forwards four times.

(ii) One-sided shrugs with wave.

Start as in exercise (i), but raise hand, wrist and arm as the shoulder circles. Keep the elbow bent. Turn the palm outwards, open out the upper chest, and at the farthest part of the circle back, wave as if to say goodbye to someone behind you (Figure 6.10). Complete the circle and repeat three to four times. Then repeat with the other arm.

Everyday benefits: More flexibility for both shoulders and rib cage, with all the improvement this brings to fuller breathing, better posture and lighter arm movements. Safer movements when driving, or when turning to look behind in any situation.

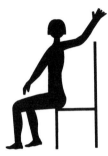

Figure 6.10

3: Hands and wrists

Sit or stand, uprightly balanced. Relax shoulders and neck, and shake the hands loosely first.

(i) Massage each hand all over with the other one, in turn. Press the thumb into the palm first and circle it with a firm pressure several times. Then massage the backs of the hands. With your thumb again, press upwards from the wrists towards and into the gaps between the fingers.

(ii) Massage each digit by pulling each firmly through the grip of the other hand several times.

(iii) Circle each finger, first freely, by itself, and then by holding it with the other hand and exploring the range of its movement.

(iv) Press each finger and thumb back in turn, first separately, and then with each digit tip to tip with its opposite number.

(v) Rotate each hand in turn, stretching and spreading the fingers like a fan. Make several turns in each direction.

(vi) Spread each hand widely and stretch its full spread. Then clench into fists and stretch again, several times.

(vii) Shake the hands loosely, both together, up and down, side to side, and round and round in both directions.

(viii) Finish with palm to palm rubs and vigorous hand-washing movements, finally encircling the wrists to complete the sequence.

4: Wrist, elbow and shoulder loosening – lying.

This very effective loosening exercise sequence draws directly on my training in Judith Aston's Fitness Programme, and I gratefully acknowledge her teaching and work.

While lying, the carriage of the head is not involved in arm movements and neck tension is avoided. Use a thin pillow, just enough to align the neck comfortably with the rest of the spine. The chin should not be tucked in or tipped back and the neck should be free. Try putting a small rolled up towel under the neck and a larger one under the waist, too, if your back arches there, for extra comfort. I sometimes close my eyes for these, to feel all the inner work going on.

Lift the right hand so that the weight of the forearm is resting vertically down through the elbow at your side. Now explore and exercise every movement that your wrist will make in this relaxed position:

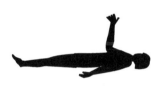

Figure 6.11

(i) Shake the hand loosely but gently, encouraging all the wrist bones to move freely (Figure 6.11).

(ii) Press the hand forwards and backwards and from side to side. Flick and then circle it round and round in each direction several times.

(ii) Let the forearm flop and fall in all directions and then circle around the elbow pivot.

(iv) Raise the arm vertically but not stiffly. Lift it and drop it back down, to feel its weight resting into the shoulder joint. Loosen the wrist (Figure 6.12).

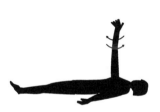

Figure 6.12

Make small circling movements in each direction, and then larger circles each way. Work slowly. Appreciate the massage going on inside the shoulder joint.

Increase the range of movement and slowly explore wherever the relaxed arm can move. Float it around in huge, nearly horizontal circles and big figures of eight, high and wide and in all directions. You should be feeling its muscular connections around the back as well as the shoulder muscles.

(v) Turn on your side with the same arm vertically up. Repeat the slow small circles and larger exploratory movements, leaning back a little to massage under the shoulder blades (Figure 6.13).

Roll on to the back, rest the right arm, and repeat the whole loosening exercise all the way from wrist to shoulder, for the left side. Rest and relax.

(vi) Now use the new suppleness of both arms together, to make fluid, creative non-symmetrical movements as if you were a ballet dancer, enjoying the lightness and flexibility of hands, wrists, elbows and shoulders (Figure 6.14). Rest and relax again.

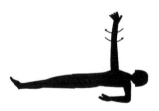

Figure 6.13

5: Opening, lengthening and releasing the hand

(i) Sit uprightly on a stool or chair with both hands hanging loosely down. First extend all the fingers lightly, then stretch them firmly down, spreading them out in the biggest possible fan. Hold for several seconds. Make tight fists and then stretch again (Figure 6.15).

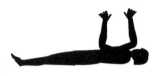

Figure 6.14

Now release most of that big stretch but continue to use enough muscle tone to let your hands stay just a little longer and more spread and open than before you stretched them. Keep this slight extra lengthening throughout the exercises.

(ii) Lift up both hands, with the fingers still lightly extended, and look at them, turning them around and getting to know them. Relax your neck, shoulders and elbows. Check that your shoulder girdle is wide and relaxed and resting lightly across your uprightly balanced spine.

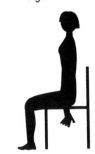

Figure 6.15

Partially rotate the hands to align the back of each with the line of the forearm. Keep the sense of relaxation and imagine them lengthening out of the wrist towards the thumb and fingertips. Widen the spread of the thumb a little. The network of muscles between the hand metatarsals is like that in the feet. The sensitivity of these muscles is enhanced as they spread and is partially lost if we screw them up (Figure 6.16). Relax and lower shoulders and elbows again.

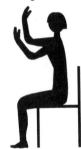

Figure 6.16

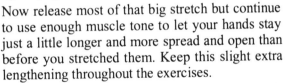

With this same alignment, rotate the forearms so that the palms face towards you and then away, alternately. Imagine that warm energy is flowing out of your hands, from the fingertips first, then out of your palms, towards you and then away.

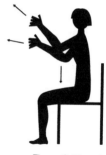

Now maintain the position with the hands facing away from you, for several seconds (Figure 6.17). Stay upright, open in the upper chest, and wide and relaxed in the shoulders, neck free, head balanced lightly. Feel the elbows weighted towards the floor and the fingertips extended with almost no ten-

Figure 6.17

sion. See if you can sense or imagine a continuing outward pressure from the palms such as healers and saints express with their hands, or we all use for receiving warmth from a fire. Tiny inner tensions will be releasing.

Next, increase your awareness of the lightness possible in your hands in movement. Soften the extension you were holding and move them around as if through water or heavy air. Float hands and arms around very lightly in all directions, shoulders open, spine lengthening up, neck and face relaxed all the time. Press them against the air as if it were a little heavier than usual, more like water (Figure 6.18).

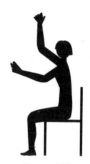

You may feel a tingling sensation that is explained in the oriental tradition as the Chi or spirit of life flowing freely in the hands and arms.

Figure 6.18

It is interesting to explore how light the hands can be in ordinary use. Lift them, palms up, turn them over, and press them lightly downwards a few times. Imagine juggling with huge light air-filled beach balls. Imagine giving and receiving a huge but weightless gift, or opening a door with hardly any effort. If you play the piano or type, imagine how light your hands and arms could be in those actions and act out some finger movements, too, almost weight-lessly floating the hands around.

The Hands at Rest

In the martial arts tradition, resting hands are never finger-linked. The specific fighting rationale for this, and for unlocked knees and free neck, too, is that in the surplus muscle effort needed to hold even a little tightness in any of these places, the body loses its readiness for action. You would have to unlink or unlock the fingers for an emergency or for fast immediate defence that was a priority in that training.

The open resting of joints and muscles is also simply the least wasteful of energy all the time, and the kindest to bodies and to ourselves. Tai Chi players rest the hands, palms up, one on top of the other, a position that can be seen in ancient pictures of Chinese sages.

Try also resting one hand palm down on your own or someone else's resting hand or arm as lightly as possible, conforming the shape to fit softly over the shape underneath. Relax elbow and shoulder and take away all surplus tension.

Benefits

These gentle hand exercises take muscle release further than usual and so help to release quite deep negative tensions such as those that we hold in tight fisted anger, disappointment and resentment.

They can also be used in a very positive way to express our spiritual good will or blessing towards the rest of the universe or the individuals we love. Even if you don't feel like a saint, you will find some interesting feelings of power available as you extend your spirit outwardly from generous well released hands.

The most ordinary actions of giving and receiving always work best when hand tensions are released. Perhaps this is the secret of the soft touch we experience with babies and small children whose way with giving and receiving has not yet acquired any psychological reservations and is sheer joy!

We know we can take in warmth from the sun or the fire, but we can also give out human warmth, comfort, acceptance and even healing. If our body, mind and spirit are open and warmly generous, other people find ways of opening up their own self healing and strength when we are with them. Humanity has these qualities plentifully if mysteriously available, operating between people, and we can find a lot of pleasure in owning them. Giving and receiving are introduced later specifically as exercises for enlivening the S-member of the B/M/S team. But the hand exercises start to give a feeling of physical extension and a practical lead to those.

EXERCISE SECTION 7

Shoulders and Neck

The Exercises

Introduction

In the previous section, the exercises for the shoulders were mostly linked with trunk, arms and hands. Here, shoulder use is related more to that of the neck and the carriage of the head.

The neck or cervical spine is part of a single linked structure, the spine. It is not a limb. It consists of the top seven vertebrae of the spine, tapering up to the skull, ahead of the locomotion and tool-wielding structures.

The top two neck vertebrae are extra special. The small atlas vertebra right at the top, at about ear level, fits with two bony rockers at the base of the skull, and enables the head to nod – see page 39. This is the nearest we come to a hinge in the whole spine. The axis vertebra below it lets the head turn from side to side, with more rotational freedom than at any other point in the spine. (To remember which of these is which, I like the phrase *Yes is higher than No.*) Together these two refinements of the spine have given land vertebrates the ability to look up, down and around to assess their environment.

Even these two specialised neck joints have only a limited range of free movement and the rest of the spine joins in when we need a bigger tilt or rotation. Don't exercise your neck as if it were attached to a rigid spine with some sort of universal joint at the top, for it is not. By treating it as a continuation of a much longer mobile structure, you will be using its mobility in the best way (Fig. 7.1).

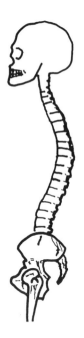

Figure 7.1. The neck is continuous with the rest of the spine. Use it with this in mind.

The exercises start with gentle rotations that involve all the spinal vertebrae, right up to the top.

The Exercises

1: Standing spinal rotations

This is a natural and relaxing movement. Children let go of tension by swinging their bodies about, and variations of this exercise are used by many therapists. Although you may have warmed up with it, use it often, and especially before the neck exercises.

Practitioners of the Bates method for improving eyesight use these rotational swings. Tai Chi players use them to promote relaxation and calm. The same exercise is also recommended for marathon runners and any whose sport involves repetitive jarring, because it helps to restore length and resilience right through the spine. It is also good after any long period of standing or sitting.

Stand with the feet apart, knees not locked. Free the neck and establish a relaxed upright balance.

Turn to one side, lift the heel of the opposite foot so that it can turn, and let the body's rotation swing the arms loosely around you (Figure 7.2).

Swing back to the other side, changing the weight and wrapping the arms the other way.

Float your head. Don't tuck the chin in tightly or tilt it up and back. Let the eyes watch their horizon all the way round — with open, not narrowed, focus — noticing everything.

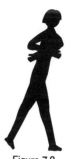

Figure 7.2

Repeat for about 30 double swings or more.

2: Neck muscle stretches

Caution

If you suffer from tension headaches, practise these gentle stretches minimally at first. If you can gradually extend the range they could help your headache problem, but do not force them.

Sitting

For all seated neck exercises, use the following alignment and relaxation details.

Sit on a firm seat, relaxed but upright. Use a stool or sit on the front edge of a chair, free to lean in all directions.

Rest hands on thighs, knees apart, elbows slightly out. Let shoulders widen and relax down. Soften the jaw, tongue, lips and eyes, your whole face open. Let the head balance lightly. Use a little abdominal tone to help to support the spine (Figure 7.3).

If possible, use a mirror to see if your torso looks balanced, open, vertical and unstrained.

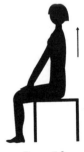

Figure 7.3

(i) Front to back

Lengthen all the way up from the sitting bones to the crown of the head. Tilt the head forwards by tipping the chin down very slightly. Now lean forwards a little, from the hips as you let your head continue to fall forwards and down. Feel a gradually increasing stretch in the muscles of the back of the neck (Figure 7.4).

Stay for a few seconds, partly supported by hands on thighs. Return slowly to the upright position, and change to a backward fall.

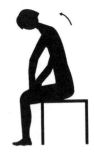

Begin to lift the chin very slowly keeping the neck long. Feel this lengthening in the sternum too, because now the whole front must lengthen.

Figure 7.4

Now slowly lean back from the hips. Let your eyes lift too, following the wall detail up to the ceiling, in a smooth and continuous line (Figure 7.5).

Don't hold this long backward lean for more than a few seconds. Return slowly, using the abdominal muscles. Notice that the neck seems a little longer and your line of sight higher than it was. Repeat the cycle front to back. Enjoy the increased length and the exercised strength of the abdominal as well as the bigger range of neck movement.

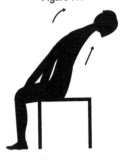

Figure 7.5

N.B: If you need to hold a backward head position, for example to study a ceiling painting, approach it in this slow and well extended way, taking frequent rests. Or find a way of resting your head on a support. Never hunch the neck back into the shoulders.

(ii) Side to side

Start by letting the head fall slightly to the left, keeping it long, the ear moving closer to the shoulder not forwards or back. Transfer your weight to the left sitting bone and let the head fall further over the left shoulder as you lean further, keeping torso as well as neck length (Figure 7.6).

Next take hold of the edge of the chair with your right hand and lean further. You should feel a distinct pull in the muscles of the right side of the neck. Hold for a few seconds and then return slowly.

Repeat to the right side. Repeat both movements.

(iii) Diagonally

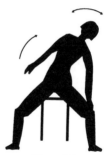

Figure 7.6

Turn your chin to the left forward diagonal. Let it start to drop as before, then lengthen and lean diagonally forwards, letting the head fall slowly forwards outside the line of the left knee. Lean till the weight of the head is felt as a heavy downward pull. Hold for a few seconds then return.

Lift up to vertical and lean slowly diagonally back to let your head fall behind you and to the right. Hold, return slowly, fully lengthened, and relax.

Repeat, making one smooth flow slowly from the forward left turn and the start of the fall, to the return back up from the backward diagonal lean. Your weight moves from one sitting bone to the other.

Turn the chin to the right corner, repeat for the right side. And repeat the whole cycle.

3: Head circles and yawns

Use a relaxed upright sitting position.

Eyes can be open or closed. Tip your nose slightly down and let the back of the neck and all of the spine lengthen up. Relax the shoulders down. Imagine a nice *right-brain friendly* image such as a flower, a smiling face or the sun, directly ahead. Then draw small imaginary circles around this picture by circling your head. If facing the sun itself, be sure to have softly closed eyelids.

Circle six times in each direction, allowing a little movement in both spine and shoulders.

Then enlarge the circle. Draw circles with the chin, your weight moving slightly from one sitting bone to the other. Circle six times each way.

Lastly, breathing fully, yawn widely and noisily and draw circles and curves in all directions with the chin. Big yawns and sighs help to release tensions of face and jaw, and, like smiling, increase the flow of blood to the brain and refresh the whole system. Yawning is good for us!

4: Head rolls, lying

Caution

For just a few people, problems with dizziness may rule out these supine head rolls. Omit them if you must, or try the first one, and gradually extend the range if your condition improves. They are wonderfully good for freeing neck and shoulders.

Lie comfortably on the mat with the thin cushion or foam pad for the head if wanted. There will be more movement for the neck if you dispense with support but choose according to your comfort.

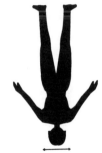

Figure 7.7

(i) First roll the head loosely and slowly from side to side, six or seven times, mouth and jaw relaxed (Figure 7.7).

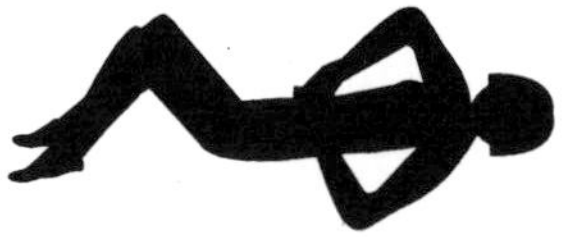

(ii) Raise the knees, a few inches apart, and clasp your hands loosely in front of the chest, palm to palm.

Roll lazily from side to side again, keeping the contact between head and mat. Roll until your nose reaches the floor, then slowly back and over to the other side. Tell your legs, body, jaw, mouth, tongue and all face muscles to relax! Imagine your eyes loose in their sockets, and even your brain loosening up inside the skull. Repeat slowly for six cycles (Figure 7.8).

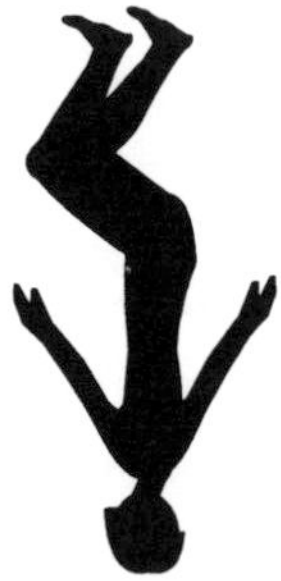

Figure 7.8

(iii) Lie with knees up and a little apart. Roll your head quite slowly to one side and knees to the other. Repeat six to eight times (Figure 7.9).

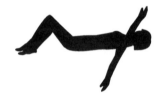

Figure 7.9

(iv) With knees raised and separated, spread the arms widely (Figure 7.10). Use four distinct and slow movements to complete this exercise:

Figure 7.10

(a) Lift the right hand and bring it loosely up and across to rest on and cup the front of your left shoulder. Watch it as it goes (Figure 7.11).

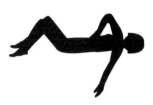

Figure 7.11

(b) Slide this hand softly along the left arm until it reaches the hand and let this movement carry the body, rolling over to the left. At the end of the roll you are lying on your left side with the fingers of the right hand touching the floor beyond those of the left (Figure 7.12). Keep the head in contact with the mat throughout.

(c) Now, slide the fingertips upwards along the floor and trace a big quarter circle until they are right above your head (Figure 7.13). Again, let your eyes follow the same route, even if you lose sight of the hand.

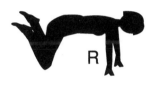

Figure 7.12

(d) While tracing this line, start to roll back, completing the fingertip semi-circle along the floor. End with arms spread and knees raised as in Figure 10.

Repeat to the right side, lifting the left hand first and following reversed steps (a) to (d) for one whole cycle. Repeat, completing four cycles in all.

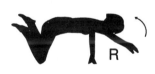

Figure 7.13

I like to add this last fluid neck and shoulder exercise sometimes to the leg and hip work in section 4, combining the two in a nicely linked exercise for the whole body in the following way.

At the end of (iv) b, (Figure 12), try extending the right leg to meet the extended right hand (Figure 7.14).

Then, at the same time as your fingers trace the semi-circle back along the floor, there comes a moment when it is easy to lift the leg high and return it to the mid line and lower it to the ground.

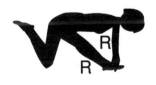

In this combined exercise, follow the foot instead of the hand with your eyes and finish as in Figure 10 again.

Figure 7.14

This may sound very athletic but it is not strenuous if you keep all the movements flowing.

Repeat for the left and once more each side.

Benefits

Neck and shoulder muscles will loosen up to carry the head more lightly. The throat becomes more open and relaxed, freeing the voice and clearing the passageways for air and nerve signals and nutrients. Your brain will be better served, and all the senses enabled to work at their best. Think about these improvements taking place. Use your newly freed voice and say openly: "That feels very, very good".

EXERCISE SECTION 8

Massage for Neck, Shoulders, Face and Scalp

The Exercises

Introduction

Faces and even scalps accumulate many tensions, and massage is a good way to help to release these. It can be delicious to have a professional facial or cranial massage, but we don't have to be massage *experts* before trying their techniques for ourselves. We can supplement a home exercise programme with massage in a quite easy *hands-on* way.

Good places to work on quite firmly are those where muscles meet the structure of the bony framework. The connective tissues here have a tendency to stiffen, especially if little used. A lighter touch is better for some of the soft and sensitive muscles especially of the face.

If you like to use a hand cream or fragrant oil, do so, but a spontaneous massage at any time will be quite comfortable with the skin just as it is. In fact, it is best not to have too slippery a surface.

The Basic Massage

Sit comfortably and reach to the bottom of the back of the neck with the finger tips of one or both hands. You can do this right now: start as far below the big vertebra at the base of the neck as you can reach, and massage firmly right up to the place where the skull rests at the top of the cervical spine, and then down again. Next work your way up and down both sides of the neck, and across the spine between the shoulder blades.

Move next to the big trapezius muscles that go from the shoulders up into the neck. Take one side at a time. Reach across with one hand to the back of the opposite shoulder and pummel and squeeze those muscles in turn. Lean your head a little towards the side you are working on to slacken the muscle as you massage it.

Next press and rub firmly all around and behind both ears with the fingertips of both hands, using small circular movements. Massage the places below and in front of the ears where the jaw articulates. Work along the lower jaw slowly and thoroughly, both along and underneath the line of the gums, and then back towards the ears. Then work down the upper jaw at gum level, and back to the hinge again.

Massage the ears themselves between fingers and thumbs. Squeeze and press the flesh and rub all over and around them. Work a little more gently forwards along the cheek bones and the sides of the nose and in a circle around the eye sockets, then quite firmly again along the line of the eyebrows, stretching the skin a little. Massage the whole forehead, making firm little circles with the fingertips, and along the hair line and around the large temple muscles high above the ears, at the sides of the scalp.

Finally plunge all of your fingers and thumbs into the hair and massage the scalp all over. Try to get some movement of the skin over the hard shell of the skull. The sensations of all these movements are pleasant. Don't rush them. You may find places that feel tighter than others, and can encourage them to recover some valuable elasticity.

A Softer Massage

After that comparatively firm and stimulating workout, or as an alternative, try a very gentle and rather different treatment for letting go. Close your eyes this time and relax into a slower and more dreamy process.

We are going to use small soft, mostly vertical little pinches, so use the tip or first knuckle of the forefinger to meet the thumb. The movements are gentle and soothing and sometimes they may release emotions that have tightened the muscles or perhaps bring back early memories from past tendernesses.

Places that respond well to this tender loving care are the big temple muscles, the forehead, the outer cheek and neck muscles and around the lower edge of the back of the skull. A *stiff upper lip* can also let go a little, and a tight jaw or locked neck can discover a softer suppleness. Any sensation of pleasure or sadness that you experience will be bringing its own inner release.

Using both hands, start between the eyebrows with small soft vertical pinches there for a few moments, and then carry the pinches slowly and softly all over brows and forehead. Next work down towards and around the front of the ears, and follow down the outer sides of the muscles of the face and cheek. This is easier to do than to describe. There is a strong masseter muscle that clamps the jaw closed and, as you soften it, it will be helped to do this job less fiercely.

Continue in along the jaw line towards the chin. Try to make tiny vertical pinches even between the lower lip and the point of the chin. Then outwards, curving up towards the ears again, and then inwards along the upper jaw line, again compressing your movements to fit some soft pinches between upper lip and the nose. Then out a little higher, at lower cheek level, and back towards the ears.

As you move to the larger muscles of the temples, scalp and sides of the neck, use more fingers for the bigger areas, but don't lose the tenderness of touch. Other candidates for this luxury are the caps of the shoulders, the upper arms, along and below the clavicles and over the central breast bone, the sternum. Treat yourself to a *tenderising* process over the surface muscles of all these areas with soft pinches or circling light finger pressure.

Once you have worked through these sequences from the text, you will automatically know how to do any future massage for these areas. The muscles remember. They enjoy it.

Benefits

Wilhelm Reich drew attention to the fact that held tension anywhere in the body involves a slight "withdrawal of the self". Eyes and faces especially reveal this habit of a slight withholding of ourselves from others. As we release these tensions we can become more open and less self-protective. We can let our natural affection and happiness show more easily. Just as all the stronger body work helps to build up self esteem, so do these gentle local releases allow for more individual and more vital expressiveness.

Massage and the Right Brain

There is a subtle creative right brain component in massage, since the sense of touch precedes language by a long way. Touch must have been the very earliest way of saying "hello"! It pre-dates words and thoughts by millions of years. So we cannot easily understand or even describe the feelings it evokes. It cannot be pinned down by explanations from the logical side of the brain.

It seems to be of the nature of muscles to respond positively to any kindly touch. Massage, brings a sense of *recognition*, an unspoken acknow-ledgement. It is as if an appreciative "Hello there!" goes positively into the nervous system, ringing bells and triggering ancient memories. When nurses in charge of premature babies have introduced deliberate stroking sessions for their tiny charges, development, even in later intelligence measurements, has been markedly advanced. Animals show the same pleasure and thriving if we have these close gentle contacts with them.

Benefits felt locally, however subtle or small, all travel right round the body, into the brain, and into nerve, hormone and immune systems too. And some of this we can easily do for ourselves with practical and simple home maintenance and caring.

Everyday Massage

When women use make-up regularly the skin benefits from the touch that these attentions involve, probably as much as from the creams or lotions we use. Men or women can do a quick *mini-facial* by taking a dry towel and rubbing very gently all around the places detailed above. We can also massage the whole scalp vigorously with the fingertips before brushing the hair, or just pinch it soothingly sometimes.

For a whole body friction-rub for the skin all over the body, it is nice to work while the skin is dry, not after a bath but before. Have a dry rub all over sometimes, morning or night, with a rough dry towel or a skin brush.

Everyday Reminders – Keep Smiling!

The exercises that are most natural to faces are yawns, smiles, kisses, laughing and singing, and lively play and conversations with friends. Cultures with very spirited ways of communication have open faces with little facial tension. If you live alone, it is a life saver to talk cheerfully to the cat, to yourself or to any imagined company! Singing and laughing are good habits for the solitary. Joining a choir is even better. Sing with the radio! Don't leave the face unexercised or tightly closed up just from being alone.

It would be nice if we still had the habit of singing at work or just exuberantly at any time, but this has almost disappeared. If someone sings in the supermarket we turn to stare! We do more listening than singing now and often spend large fortunes on it. But wonderful as that may be, we should avoid becoming listeners only! Make a point of finding imaginative ways to lessen the effects that social conventions and restrictions can have on any of our muscles, and minds and spirits too, for these are all meant to be expressively free.

The tension release that massage brings can help to stimulate a more expressive use of face and voice, and greater awareness as well as aliveness for eyes and mind, body and spirit, at all times. There may seem to be only a minor surface improvement from this little massage exercise, but little by little you will come to value this extra release.

Yawn and stretch when you wake up in the morning. Think your way round the face muscles while still in bed and let night time tensions go. We often tense the jaw or forehead in our sleep. Think your way along some of these muscles and soften the eyes and let go of the dreams or anxieties or the habits of tension before you get up. It will be easier to give the day a really warm, welcoming, wholehearted yawn and stretch.

EXERCISE SECTION 9

Ways of Relaxing and Releasing

The Exercises

Introduction

These are ways of putting the principles of openness and lengthening and expansion into the purpose of deep release and restoration. As exercises they should be entered into awarely, noticing those principles in action.

The benefits of relaxation are very like those of physical exercise. The muscle release they encourage lowers the levels of blood sugar and adrenaline which become raised under emotional and psychological, as well as bodily or nutritional stress. Any of these stresses can undermine our fitness at any time. It is rare for any of us today to avoid them completely, and rest and recovery from them is absolutely necessary to our health.

Everything in the living body works with a balance of exertion and rest, and, important as plentiful activity is, the resting period of this cycle is as essential as the working one. Cells alternately work and recover. Muscles alternately contract and release. The diaphragm, heart, other muscles and lungs all work with a natural cycle of work/relax. In our bi-pedal walking, the muscles of one leg work to propel us and then relax while the other one takes over. All the way from small scale rests at the cellular level, right up to short holiday breaks or a long convalescence, or even sometimes a month at the seaside, we need our breaks for rest. Try to find time for at least 10-20 minutes of positive recuperative relaxation every day, perhaps in two separate and different sessions of letting go.

Fine Tuning

We can experience physical tension at several levels. A tightly clenched fist or jaw is visibly tense and we can see when it relaxes. But deeper tensions can be invisible yet very persistent.

When we carry deeply accumulated tension patterns around, they block our sensitivity. They are like armour. We lose touch with our real needs, and with our intrinsic inner optimism and vitality. We may live our lives almost one step away from the reality of what matters to us. We don't even notice our need to rest! We can become workaholics, or eat and drink inappropriately or adopt other self destructive habits.

When we do let go of stored tension patterns, we are able to listen more sympathetically to the body, and to our inner good sense, and even more sensitively to each other. Our choices and priorities about work, food, responsibilities and fun, as well as rest, can all clarify. In fact, a very good time to make important choices is immediately after a period of deep relaxation when body, mind and spirit have settled into a more whole integration.

Here are five ways of relaxing/releasing, giving plenty of variety. Experiment with them. They include lying, sitting, standing, moving and, lastly, a process of inner relaxation that can become an inner healing journey.

Horizontal Relaxing

This is a very well known, basic process. The detail given is simply in the interest of raising awareness. It will soon become a pleasure to run through all of these small steps, almost automatically.

Lie down with enough support for the head to maintain the natural curve of the neck without stress. Tuck a small folded towel there for extra comfort if you like. Check that your head is free to rotate and to nod slightly, neither tilted back nor tucked tightly down. A few tiny nods and shakes will quickly undo any neck lock. The larynx should not feel squashed or the teeth clamped. The supply channels of the throat need to be well open always to serve both body and brain. Use a light blanket for warmth if needed.

One of the most relaxing positions for the spine is with the knees raised and feet a little apart, a position recommended in the Alexander Technique. Or lie with legs well extended if you prefer. If you want to rest for a longer time have the legs also apart, and perhaps use small soft cushions or rolled towels under the knees to help the muscles to let go. A smaller pad could go under the mid-back, adjusted to fill any small gap there. Especially if the spine is stiff, these gentle supports can be comforting and comfortable muscles more easily let go. It is fine to use this relaxation process in bed if the mattress is moderately firm and the covers light and loose.

Begin by deliberately letting go of all worries. Stop judging yourself or anyone else. Imagine the universe getting on very well without you, other people doing what they are doing, and having whatever opinions and feelings and desires they are having too. The universe can manage perfectly well for a short time without your comments and anxieties and assessments!

The delicious sense of well earned rest will deepen. Listen to your breathing as it slows down and expands. Imagine the whole torso breathing, from the shoulders right down to the perineum. The ribs can press down against the mat at your back, and out to the sides, too. As you inhale or exhale, imagine breath flowing all through the body as if your limbs were hollow. Send it all the way to the finest capillaries of toes and finger tips, and out through the pores of the scalp.

This is a good time for experiencing your length and width. Imagine the central axis of the spine to be gradually releasing into its fullest possible length, all the way up. Don't try to push anything, but imagine all the partnerships along it opening out to their fullest width. Your back broadens and the front widens; shoulders widen and hip bones move subtly apart. Even the kidneys move further apart. Lungs and rib cage widen and relax down towards the floor. Jaws, cheeks, eyes and nostrils soften and widen. The two hemispheres of the brain relax and expand in the roominess of the skull. A sort of inner spreading goes on as all your length and width claim their full space in the world.

Now consciously welcome your own powers of restoration which you know to be naturally strong. Put them in touch with some universal healing magic, too, and invite them to get on with their good work. Then switch off and just rest while this restoration goes on. Ten to 15 minutes will be enough if this is a daily rest. Stay longer if you feel particularly in need. Then roll over, rise refreshed and enjoy whatever activity comes next. A longer inner journey will be described later.

Standing Relaxing

Check alignment first and relax into an easy, standing uprightness. Have the feet a little wider than hip width apart, evenly grounded, knees relaxed, head lightly balanced. Don't bend forwards, lean or arch your back from hips, waist, at upper chest or neck. Avoid the little forward lift of the chest we sometimes adopt when wanting to stand up straight. We want good front length but not a forward thrust or military style importance.

Your foot sensors can give information about leaning. Lean back on the heels until nearly too far. Lean forwards on to the transverse arch until you know it is carrying more than its share. Try a sideways lean. Circle your weight round as you try out the limits of the foot support and then choose a balance between them. If you lift the toes momentarily and press down across the ball of the foot, the abdominal support will reward you with a little more muscle tone and your front length may increase. This small check can be a useful reminder at other times. It prevents us from leaning over the knees and helps towards a good alignment.

Relax the shoulders out and down while the neck lengthens up from between the shoulder blades. A very slight lowering of the nose or chin can help the spine to lengthen up, but not so far that the teeth touch or clench or the voice box feels squashed. Relax hands, jaw, neck, mouth and eyes, and rest uprightly. Don't try too hard with any of these pointers but think around each as you get ready to put your anti-gravity system in charge.

Relax thighs and buttocks. Don't tuck the seat tightly under or push it back. Release the sitting bones downwards. Allow the breath to slow down and to expand you lightly.

Now close your eyes without lowering them and imagine yourself in a nice place, at a beach, forest, waterfall or somewhere you love to be, and imagine a feast of wonderful sounds, sights and scents. Rest in this position for several minutes, keeping a sense of extension upwards and 3-D expansion all over. Imagine yourself expanding fully and easily and claiming your personal, rightful share of space in this blissful scene.

Sitting Relaxing

Zen and other forms of meditation use variations of the sitting position. The version I choose here uses a firm kitchen or dining chair without arms, or a stool to sit on, which is easier for many people than a cross-legged position or sitting back on the heels on the floor. You need the sitting bones as a firm base, so don't slump into your favourite armchair. Imagine your torso is *standing* uprightly on these bones. Sit with your weight back where the spine is. Have knees apart, lower legs relaxed, vertical or almost so, the weight of the knee over the arch of the foot. Spread the feet to feel the floor, then relax them in comfortable contact with it.

Keep the upper chest wide open, the whole rib cage very slightly lifted out of the waist, and let the abdominal muscles come naturally into use. Your weight will be both settling down on the sitting bones, and also rising up along the spine towards the sky. Try to direct in both directions at once.

Widen the shoulders and release them down, both at the sides and the back, so the main weight of the arms is carried on the strongly vertical spine via the shoulder yoke. Rest your hands lightly on the thighs, wrists and fingers released from tensions.

Close the eyes, relax jaw, mouth, tongue and eyes, and stay in this position for several minutes. Use a fraction of your attention to keep checking postural points, lengthening up, and releasing local tensions from the body and face, or anxieties from the mind if they arise. This focusing of attention is not hard work and is a part of the letting go process. Sit for about 10 minutes like this before opening the eyes and carrying on with the day's work and play.

Moving Relaxation

It is very refreshing to relax in movement. Many cultures use dance, slow walking or whirling or even fast running as traditional activities of special significance, like a meditation. For some of us dancing or jogging are very good ways of releasing tension, but for others, especially as we grow older, these can introduce bodily strains we don't want. The free and relaxed movements that children use, like rolling on the ground or swinging the arms might be even better if we could feel comfortable with them. This moving relaxation process derives from the oriental martial arts tradition. It borrows their principle of complete relaxation in movement without the detailed structure of specific forms.

Music helps bodies to relax, just as it helps us to march or to dance even when tired. Play a tape of favourite music that is *right-brain friendly* and not too demanding, or sing or hum your own songs. Don't choose music that is artificially synthesised, or has a strong beat or a very repetitive form, because we want to let go of all left brain controls. Pleasurable, non-taxing, musical sounds help the right brain to encourage physical and emotional release. They will contribute to holistic repair and healing if we open up to them. Humming is said to loosen even scalp tightnesses. Give yourself some musical extras as a treat sometimes. Even if you feel sceptical about this process, try putting all scepticism on one side and just play with this moving relaxation, if only ever once, as an interesting releasing exercise.

Start by standing still with eyes closed. Relax any noticeable tensions of neck face hands and shoulders. Then simply begin to move. At first respond to whatever impulse comes, or to the music. If you feel like scratching your knee or massaging a stiff shoulder, do that. Or stretch your fingers, circle the head or change your weight from one foot to the other. Then let slow movements simply follow one another, arms, head and feet moving in non-symmetrical ways. This is not the same as dance. Don't try to act or be expressive of anything other than the fact that bodies are revitalised by flowing unforced movement, and are able to move well even without seeing. Another time, you could use similar movements to create some more expressive dancing, but that would be a different exercise.

Just explore slow movements for themselves: wide stretches, small hand movements, high reaches and low squats too, quite slowly, feeling each one awarely. If you share with a partner you can take turns to protect one another from bumping into anything, and use bigger steps and bolder sweeps of the arms.

Five minutes of the concentration of this moving relaxation goes quickly but your body will feel its effects for a long time afterwards. There is something about the eyes-closed condition, removing some of the major references for balance, that compels the proprioceptive system to work from its inner signals only. The memory of that feeling of an inner connected wholeness stays with us. It can remind the body at other times of the pleasures that belong in movement itself, and it will grow more confident in its natural balance and other skills.

I remember a similar lasting effect from skiing down a long mountain run once in the dark in an Inner Game exercise. The ski run was familiar and there was a very faint light from the moon, but still my feet and legs had to feel for gradients and bumps and respond with very few visual clues. It was extraordinarily liberating and lasting in its pleasure.

Inner Relaxation and Inner Healing

The first time you try this inward exploratory relaxation process, lie comfortably and settle down to it as an extension of the first method above. As you grow familiar with it, you could fit it, or small parts of it into any time of day.

Again, the description seems to take a long time, but after the first time we can draw on its benefits quite speedily, whether lying, sitting, standing or walking.

The inner journey you take for this relaxation can be abbreviated, lengthened or speeded up. It makes a good start to the day, in bed before getting up, or a good finish before sleep at night. When we are not feeling well it encourages a profound rest that speeds the healing. It is a visualisation in which your positive imagination acknowledges and appreciates all your body, all its processes and all it is doing to support you. Allow 20 minutes first time.

Start by imagining that you are exploring inside the palms of both hands, encouraging them to feel warmer and very open. Usually they will soon feel physically warmer, but even imagined warmth is fine. Then imagine that you are exploring further inside, and keep going. Go from the palms up through the thumbs and each finger of both hands together. Admire all that you see in there even if there are trouble spots and encourage any of these to get better quickly. Work your way around all the bones and ligaments and blood vessels of the hand, then back into the wrists.

Imagine plenty of space everywhere on this inner journey: open passageways, non-squashed nerves and healthy blood vessels all free to carry information and nutrients most efficiently. Work your way around the muscles of the forearms, through the elbow joints, up to the upper arms and all around and through the shoulder joints. Visualise smooth healthy muscles everywhere, bright nerves and blood vessels, shiny sinews, strong bones meeting in smooth efficient joints. Watch very pure blood surging along, and high-speed electric signals pulsing through nerves, a lively pageant of active good health throughout the whole body.

You need not consciously relax. Muscle release will be going on. It is your acknowledgement and appreciation of this inner space and teamwork that encourages release. Think of giving three-dimensional space and perfect health to all the mechanisms, fluids, tubes and joints while you admire them. It will help if you gradually make an increasingly accurate acquaintance with your anatomy. Take a look at the skeleton of a hand sometimes, or the position and shape of your inner organs. The more you can visualise the detail of joints and organs the better.

Keep going! Widen and relax the shoulders as you visit them, then go along both clavicles and into the rib cage, as if into a big wide barn or engine room. There is a lot happening in here. Stand inside that cavity and appreciate its spaciousness. Admire the way your lungs and the big muscle of the heart pulse life around. Admire the complexity of it all. Imagine your breath filling the whole torso, expanding the space so that every organ has plenty of room and operates at its best. See your heart pumping healthy nutrients and oxygen to the farthest extremities, and if there are unwell places, encourage the whole team to bring support for their special needs.

Notice your ribs widening out and closing in, rhythmically and easily. Feel their pressure against the support beneath you too. To include your spirit, make contact with the universe outside as well, and see your own private inner oneness in that bigger context of everything else.

Don't feel separate from the natural or man-made world but part of everything that is. Keep breathing in fresh healing energy as if from the whole generous world outside you, using heart and lungs together as joint centres of vitality, love, positive energy and healing. Having drawn in magically from the environment with every breath, these strong pumps are busy sending new life and healing to every part of you. You can extend their vitality with some goodwill of your own that can travel outside, to people and worlds far away across all boundaries and to the other side of all universes.

As the lungs act so clearly as our interface with the universe we can imagine them as a sort of placenta. Universal nourishment flows into them from outside, as if with maternal generosity, all the time. Then the heart takes over, draws from the reservoir of the lungs, and pumps this freely given vitality around inside you, delivering universal health and healing with every heart beat. Remember that images do not have to be real to be of great value. You might choose to imagine a big team of medical helpers, or living cells acting like factory workers all buzzing with positive activity. Just make every inner image a positive and supportive one. Perhaps that is what the imagination is for!

This is a time to think about living in a maximally healthy way and using your particular supports, aids and beliefs, in the area of healing. If you have a special support system or belief pattern use it now. It will be right for you. But if you have been sceptical about any kind of *faith* aspect to healing, just recognise that all the healing that ever goes on in your body is done by you! Where other people make a special contribution, whether doctor or healer, it is always in awakening your own inner abilities that are already there, whether with medicine, bedside care, laying on of hands or even witch doctoring.

Inner positive work (or play) with your own imagination can help you to take over some of this restorative power. As long as you choose to give space to your own positive intentions for fitness, you will be opening up the possibilities of your own expanding health.

Try to visit all the organs, every cell, the tiniest blood vessels and nerves. Give each one plenty of space. Release any little tensions around them. Watch the way in which they all know exactly what to be doing and how to adjust moment by moment to changes in the demands or the sudden needs of all the others. Visit your stomach, liver, intestines, as if you were watching a television screen. See everything working well for you. Keep exploring around like a visitor in a science or engineering museum! You can visit the glands of your endocrine system, the genitals, reproductive organs, bladder and colon and all the orifices and sphincters. Admire the good work and expert functioning everywhere, inviting improvement anywhere it may be needed.

Then leave the complex torso and visit the locomotion department. Send your attention down the big muscles of the front of the thighs. Admire their resting potential and strength. If they feel tight, ask them to relax for you. Explore inside the knees, and down the fronts of the lower legs, ankles, feet and toes, round under the toes and to the soles of the feet where you can pause and generate warmth again. Return via the heels, the back of ankles, calves, knees, leg and the power house of the buttock muscles.

On this return walkabout take in the joints of the hips, pelvis and sacrum, the kidneys and all the spine. Imagine them healthy and free. Explore nerves and channels, every joint and spinal vertebra, and the spinal chord, well fortified inside its smooth white canal. It can be a fascinating journey. There are clean, shiny cartilage surfaces, and plump healthy discs between the spinal vertebrae topping up with fresh fluids and lubricants. While you are resting and admiring them, trace these nicely cushioned vertebrae one by one, all the way up to the base of the skull. Watch repair work going on if bones are worn, muscle fibres torn or tiny blood vessels constricted.

When you arrive at the neck, the cervical spine, make a sortie into your throat and explore the special openness here. Go in and around the oesophagus, trachea and voice box. Notice how wonderfully well all this equipment is, how open, clean, clear and unsquashed, and how fantastically well it works for you. Promise it some good conditions as you see it all in action. You will realise at first hand how open it likes to be.

Move up into the big cave of the mouth, and around the teeth and into the jaw and its hinges. Notice your tongue, a big soft muscle resting in its warm moist environment, relaxed and waiting until you need it again. Let your mouth fill with saliva as you relax it, and taste this as healthy and sweet and nourishing.

Explore the open and clear labyrinths of the ears too, and the channels of the nose and sinuses. Feel your eyes floating and relaxed in their sockets. Move them around a little and then rest them again. Inside the brain, watch the elaborate network of nerves and brain cells. They are working brilliantly. See that the two big hemispheres have plenty of space and are relaxed, with plenty of room, cooperating happily.

Enjoy this visit to your brain. It will be happy to have you as a visitor. There is so much to marvel at. Admire the visual cortex, the memory centres, the language department and other places so complex that we may never fully understand them. See them relaxed and efficient, helpful and comfortable, in spacious surroundings, handling millions of processes brilliantly while you are looking on. See the brain as very fit, doing a perfect job and managing some admirable teamwork.

The cooperation going on in brain and body alike could be a model for any society! Everything seems to know what everything else needs, and is keen to supply its part of that need. Blood vessels bring oxygen and nutrients along exactly as required, and you can promise the whole system the very best conditions you can provide.

See that every artery and vein is clean and roomy inside. Sweep or ream them out if they seem to need a spring clean. Finally, observe appreciatively that memory, eyesight, hearing – all your sensing apparatus, is in excellent shape. Slip round between the brain and the skull and between the skull and the scalp, and around your skin all over the body, and declare your journey complete.

Peter Schellenbaum introduces this process, as an *inner massage* and calls it a way of "practising attentiveness to the body". His special use is to recommend it as a way of relaxing from a basic existential problem that leaves its traces in all human beings. No infant ever feels that it is loved as totally as it was in the womb, and we can carry these feelings of existential disappointment as a sort of perceived insufficiency of love, right into our adulthood. An appreciative inner excursion, he says, can help to put us back into our own lives more centrally as we take over the providing of some of our own inner caring and acknowledgement.

Many therapists use variations of this exercise, using awareness of the body as a way into other levels of awareness, psychological and spiritual, too. I see it as one that will work its magic for us wherever we choose to put our attention with total acceptance and positive appreciation. If you are looking for bodily relaxation and healing, that will be its major benefit for you. If you are willing to release psychological and emotional tensions at the same time, they will find ways of evaporating too. And if you wish to observe a spiritual part of your selfhood operating and extending beyond the body and mind, this extra linkage will be there, too, in the images you create for this bigger extension of yourself.

Conscious Coordination –
Important Linkages for Body and Brain

Introduction

The coordination exercises of this section strengthen linkages across the two sides of the body and they are valuable for this alone. But they also challenge the corresponding nerve linkages across the brain.

They put to practical use the fact that the left brain manages movement in the right side of the body and vice versa. Coordinated left/right movements automatically stimulate cooperation across the two brain hemispheres as well as warming up the muscles. They are very easy to do and, even if you are well coordinated, worth doing as an energising tonic for muscles and nerves. If you know your coordination is poor you need them more, but in this case, stick to the simplest, do them often, and always very slowly.

The Upright Quadruped

We know that muscle imbalance happens rather easily in the human biped. Instead of an even tone all over, some muscles may become too tense while others become too slack. Because of the way muscle linkages spiral round the structure, even a small rotation, minor bend or lean or thrust becomes easily reinforced and gradually more pronounced.

This imbalance is much less likely to happen in a quadruped and the coordination exercises are reminders to our muscles and nerves of the beautifully balanced pattern of animal movement that we inherit from quadrupeds.

Dr Janet Goodrich has called the basic cross-crawl coordination exercise *brain surgery,* to make its brain and vision benefits more vivid, and she strongly recommends it in her teaching. She likens a poor or unpractised cooperation between the brain hemispheres to a partial or total *switching off* of the connection between them, so that one side comes to be dominant. These are good images to use. There is no mechanical switch, of course, and no surgeon's knife. But a few easy, coordinated movements can be seen as pushing messages along neglected pathways. We can imagine this having the effect of keeping open, opening up more clearly or actually *switching on* the tired linkages across the two sides.

I see this exercise also as one that brings us into the present moment, persuading body and mind to be in the same place at the same time. This is always a force for good.

Keeping Brain Linkages Open

Cross-crawl exercises have been used therapeutically to help people with minor dyslexia problems and other difficulties in mental organisation. People with such problems are often very creative. A little work to improve physical coordination can help to turn a disorganised creativity into a much more effective and practical one. If you have a severe problem you will need specialist help, but for our minor problems of everyday mental disconnectedness, cross-crawl can be a very helpful tool.

While doing these exercises keep your attention on the two opposites you are working with. Sometimes it will be hand and opposite foot. But elbow to knee or hand to knee and many other cross over connections can be used. Keep in mind, too, the opening up of all the many channels of cross connection that are under-used in many of our bi-pedal activities.

The Exercises

1. Basic Cross-Crawl Movements

Begin by making loose fists with both hands. Then lift the right fist and the left knee forward and up as if marching, but more freely than a march. By softening the movements the hand action need not be rigidly tied to that of the foot. If you watch a quadruped closely its walk is not like clockwork (Figure 10.1).
Repeat for left fist and right knee.

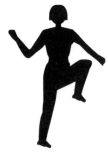

Figure 10.1

Keep alternating these movements slowly and rhythmically for a few minutes, or longer. Use the flexibility of the feet and ankles to keep your step light and springy. Balance the head lightly and relax tension in the limbs. It is not a goose step or military march. If the coordination slips, stop and start again.

For most of us this basic exercise comes easily, and we can add any of the variations below. If you find the basic one at all difficult omit the variations below and just work with basic cross-crawl. You can add variations one by one as coordination improves. It will improve if you take the movements slowly and reinforce this exercise with all the loosening up work, yawning and relaxation, and persist with the basic practice.

Cross-crawl can also be done sitting. Odd moments in the car or watching television can be used for this. Use small inconspicuous movements if you don't want to have to explain yourself to inquisitive friends.

Variation 1
Walk or skip, perhaps sing with cross-crawl or some of its variations or do them to music. We are designed to move exuberantly, not always in studied and serious actions, and free movement and cheerful music enliven the right brain. But even if you sing and dance, keep your attention on the two opposite limbs, or parts of them that you are involving together.

2: Diagonal stretches

Extend the right hand high up, forward and to the right, and the left leg out widely and back to the left. Deliberately stretch fingers and toes. Then reach the opposite way and keep alternating the movements. This one does not lend itself to a very fast version (Figure 10.2).

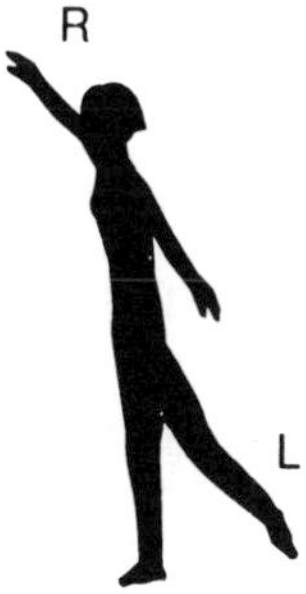

R

L

Figure 10.2

3: Swinging walking

With upright posture, walk forwards, lifting up the left knee and swinging the right arm high up towards the sky, and then the right knee and the left arm. Alternate these movements as you walk.

Use pauses if you lose the coordination. If it is easy, move continuously and rhythmically (Figure 10.3).

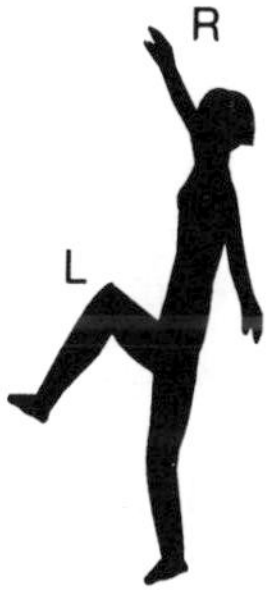

R

L

Figure 10.3

4: Knee and elbow out

Turn the left knee out widely to the left, and raise the right elbow out to your right side (Figure 10.4). Reverse the position and repeat several times.

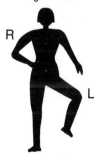

R

L

Figure 10.4

5: Elbow to opposite knee

Swing the right elbow across you to meet the raised left knee, and alternate this movement. Try not to hunch up. If they don't meet, the gap does not matter (Figure 10.5).

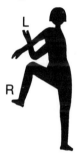

L

R

Figure 10.5

6: Kick back crossover

Reach behind you with the right hand and kick the left heel up and back towards it (Figure 10.6).

Reverse the position, kicking back the right foot and meeting it, (or not quite) with the left hand.

Repeat many times, slapping at the heels alternately.

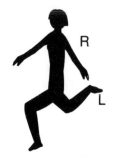

Figure 10.6

7: Hand to opposite knee

Slap the raised left knee with partly cupped right palm, and then the right knee with left palm. Repeat and continue alternating these movements (Figure 10.7).

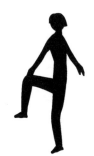

Figure 10.7

8: Hand to opposite foot

Kick the left leg high in front and circle the extended right arm back and right round before reaching across towards the left toes with the fingers of the right hand. Keep the back long. Use big movements. Don't curl up. You don't have to touch if you cannot reach (Figure 10.8).

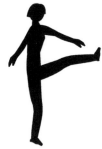

Figure 10.8

Everyday Opportunities

Bring a cross-energy awareness to ordinary walking sometimes, as an exercise. Try carrying a back-pack instead of a briefcase or shopping bag, to free shoulders and arms to swing. Sometimes emphasise the swing of elbow or shoulder to keep the mental linkage alive.

Stay awake to the use of the eyes, too, for visual benefits from cross-crawl movements. Trace your vision round the outlines of buildings, trees and landscape while walking, so that vision has to use its complex cross linkages. Keeping visually alert is part of our holistic aliveness and helps to strengthen the wide awakeness of the brain and the whole person.

Don't struggle with these exercises. Your left brain can try too hard. Struggle increases tension and that depletes energy and upsets coordination, and will add to rather than reduce tiredness. Done lightly, they are all energising and excellent for clearing fatigue, irritation, and other accompaniments of tension in body or mind.

Supine cross-crawling

This exercise can be done in bed before getting up in the morning, a good time to be switching on. Sitting or lying it can be done to wake you up at any time.

Have the feet wide apart at first and hands well separated above your head to lengthen the body.

If you are doing this exercise in bed, try pushing back the pillow and letting it rest on your up-turned palms, with shoulders released and wide. Your hands will relax more openly under the light weight of the pillow.

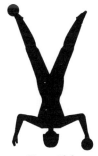

Begin the exercise by tightening all the fingers of the left hand, and all the toes of the right foot, together. Then relax these and pause.

Next tighten the opposite pair: right fingers and left toes together. Relax and pause. Repeat this movement many times, omitting the pauses as it becomes easy (Figure 10.9).

Figure 10.9

You will need to keep your attention in the extremities being exercised to prevent slipping into a one-sided mode. If you do find that right fingers and right toes are tightening together, stop and start again.

Variation 1

Try flexing just your right thumb and left big toe, and then the left thumb and right big toe. Do this several times. Then move to curl or press down the index finger with second toe of the opposite foot, and work very slowly in turn with third fourth and fifth digits.

Variation 2

Bring the feet close together and hands close together till touching, and repeat any of these variations.

Relax briefly after any session of cross-crawl exercises. See if you can detect next time you do the exercise that positive changes have taken place in your coordination. Imagine that you can also sense a new ability to handle problems and projects more confidently, because the mental spin-off is always consolidated more easily if we look for it. And then specifically acknowledge those benefits, however small.

The switched on time after cross-crawl is a good moment for making decisions and also for making healthily positive affirmations about your whole general B/M/S fitness. "Things are getting better and better in my fitness and my life, day by day". You can decide to build on your increasing fitness now and feel optimistic about the way your life is going forward, more awarely and more positively.

A one-minute refresher for body and mind

If you feel bored, do 10 (or 16, 20, 30 or more) of any of the crossover exercises above or any you can invent, in cheerful spontaneous succession. A variety is probably better than just one, though for people with a coordination problem, one minute of the basic cross-crawl would be a better choice.

Ten of each of the following can easily fit into a minute or two:

❐   Basic cross crawl

❐   Diagonal stretches

❐   Swing walking

❐   Elbow crossing to opposite knee

❐   Kick back crossovers

❐   Slap right knee with left palm, and vice versa.

Don't stand and slump while the microwave heats a cup of coffee or you boil an egg. One or three whole minutes can be spent really valuably in this way and can restore flagging energy at any time.

If you are sitting, there are several varieties that you can adapt for a similar refresher. Pressing down opposite little finger and opposite little toe a few times can be quite a challenge.

When to use cross-crawl movements

I like to use cross-crawl, or sometimes a whole Tai Chi form, specifically to help with complex decision making or in preparation for a difficult task. Confusion and disorder often indicate some lack of cooperation between different departments in the brain. My rational and creative selves can be in opposition or wanting several quite different things at once!

Bringing physical connectedness can be the beginning of very fruitful and purposeful creativity. Confusion is not necessarily a negative state. Plenty of good ideas are buzzing round when we are confused, but with encouragement they can take shape as a coherently brilliant plan.

Another use is in bringing the rational mind to help sort out an irrational emotion and allow common sense to come back to an upsetting situation when it may have left the scene and abandoned you to rage or gloom. Just making the pause to do some cross-crawl has benefits for the thinking departments and can open up possibilities for taking a new look.

Faced with a problem that seems too complex, take time first to think about the many practicalities involved in it however various and muddled they seem. Perhaps write some of them down in a list for a better look at them, or spread them around a page loosely grouped and linked as Tony Buzan recommends. Then stop worrying and do several minutes of coordination exercises. (If that seems like a war dance, don't worry! Witch doctors were probably clearing their minds too!) Go back to the problem and tackle one small manageable part of it, and order will begin to appear.

Going for a walk when that is possible makes a good cross-crawl interlude. You may well find that a new idea or new clarity emerges from the complexity and that you feel able to trust a new decision or produce a master plan. The musician Roberto Gerhard did much of his composing walking round the streets and gardens of Cambridge. Many creative people spontaneously walk to clear the head and let the ideas take shape.

During and after these movements the brain starts to tackle problems afresh and transform disorder into order, or vague ideas into good ones, step by practical step. It is one of the claims of Tai Chi practice, that it clears the mind for the next decision or the next step to be taken. And Tai Chi shares this cross energy emphasis, using the limbs very consciously. In all Tai Chi practice, while the left leg is firmly rooted it is the right hand that is *active*.

Perhaps brain surgeons will one day do some fancy bypass operations across the corpus callosum and keep the two sides of the human biped's brain permanently operating in equal partnership! Meanwhile this on-the-spot *brain surgery*, whatever you think about it, can be your own effective DIY operation at times when you feel unbalanced, *switched off*, disorganised or low in energy. Even if you treat it as a little ritual or placebo, the exercise will work towards clarification and the summoning of energy to act.

Our assorted patterns of disconnectedness are very individual. Of course, we cannot handle very severe ones by movement alone, and you may not produce a symphony each time you go for a walk! But you will come to know when cross-crawl can help clear the mind in situations of minor disorientation or muddle, and then you will put it to regular use. The physical benefit of improved bodily coordination and balanced muscle use is, in any case, enough reason to include these exercises in every home exercise repertoire.

Walking: The Upright Quadruped Steps Out

When it comes to ordinary everyday walking, both the animal quadruped in us and the newer, human biped are in operation, and I believe we should not exaggerate either mode. We should neither overemphasise the four-limbed involvement of cross coordination, – except when exercising to remind ourselves, nor swing too deliberately from side to side as skaters must.

Skaters are very bi-pedal. They have no friction between foot and ground to help forward propulsion and no heel-toe action available either. They have to throw all the body's weight from foot to foot for really fast action, *tacking* along instead of taking the body's axis straight ahead.

Somewhere between these extremes of four-limbed crossover connectedness and a strictly bi-pedal locomotion, there is a free and natural walk that is just right for the individual you.

Our posture is unique to us and our walk is our very own, too. See that there is some lift, not a slump in your step in order to carry your weight up not down, and lightly not heavily from foot to foot. Let some of the energy of the forward swing of each arm find its way into the whole forward movement, so that it helps to carry your vertical axis forwards.

Like the horse, for which walking, trotting, cantering and galloping all use the limbs in slightly different ways, our walk is also changeable and complex. But we can think of the light swing of the arms as contributing forward momentum for the top half of the body. It cannot heave you up much from a shuffle or slump. But if you are up the unforced momentum of its natural swing can give a little kick to the forward propulsion, high above the ground, just at that lightest moment at the top of the rise.

The human biped can walk or skate perfectly well with hands behind our backs or stiffly beside us, using our two legs and nothing else. But our whole body really likes to be part of our purposeful forwardness, and that means all four limbs are involved.

Experiment sometimes. Notice and exaggerate the distinct two-sidedness. Notice and exaggerate the four limbs cooperating. Try some very slow walking and some backward walking. When very slow we can feel one whole side carrying the weight of the head first, and then the other side takes over. As we speed up our forward walk, the extra forward momentum smoothes out this side-to-side component into a straight-ahead progress. The feet will be wider apart if very slow and will fall almost in line for very fast running.

So what guidelines can we use every day when we inherit such adaptability and huge scope? All the basic considerations still apply. The body should be upright and lengthening up, the shoulders wide and across the spine to carry the arms lightly. The mid-section should be long and well toned. And there should be an upward anti-gravity springiness and forward momentum to help carry the body along during the weight changes from foot to foot.

We should avoid a clockwork or goose-step mechanism or rigid arm swing. A smooth one limb at a time process operates subtly if we remove tensions and excessive control. Competitive walking or the exaggerated arm work as used for taxing the body in a cardiovascular workout, have some value but put a big strain on the body. If you do these, loosen and stretch afterward to stay limber. We should avoid special effects if we are no longer young and have long-term maintenance in mind.

The loosening up exercises throughout this programme help us to stay supple enough to be able to let go of any hard work in our ordinary everyday walking. Then more of the energy of our direction and purpose, and of each limb, goes simply into mechanically smooth propulsion.

EXERCISE SECTION 11

Exercises for The Mind and Mental Awareness

The Exercises

Visualisation and Affirmations

A primary mental exercise is that of simply focusing our fullest attention on any activity at any time and doing it extremely well with heart and mind and spirit. This active cooperation, mind and body coming together in the here and now, always absorbs, refreshes and enlivens us. Any of the bodywork exercises, done awarely, help to make us more alert mentally as well as fitter physically. And the cross crawl group especially make a definite contribution to mental clarity and balance.

But there are other more specific exercises we can use. In this section we explore the well accepted mind techniques of *visualisation* and of making *affirmations*. These are two psychological techniques that recruit the mind into the world of training for practical and behavioural skills. Each is popular and used effectively in both sports and business trainings. Skills that successful psychologists coaches and trainers have pioneered and use widely with good results, can be equally valuable to us in ordinary everyday home fitness work.

The Imagination as a Positive Ally

Other animals may also have the beginnings of inner pictures and dreams, but human minds have a unique ability to imagine very vividly and to express their imaginings in words. We can summon up mental pictures of objects, events, movements, skills – all manner of things. We can remember events from long ago in great detail. We can dream, wish, fantasise and turn dreams into works of art or practical adventures. Our imagination is a wonderfully important human gift and one to use and enjoy. Imagining becomes an exercise when we take time to direct it purposefully towards a specific outcome or a definite improvement we want to make.

With a little practice we can train our imagination to be more positively supportive than it is now, of our health, vitality and our unique way of life. The secret is that the more positively we use it the better it will serve us as long as we are also doing practical things to reach the same goal and are not just hoping and wishing. We can polish its positive skills

A good mental exercise at any time is simply to turn mentally towards a positive direction; to switch to plus. We can *think plus* or, better still, *speak plus*, and then go a step further and *do something plus*. Professional trainers, when they use techniques of visualisation and spoken affirmations, are building on this basic exercise for the mind and the imagination. They know how powerful positive images can be. They will use them along with other exercise schedules to make positive goals come to life for their trainees.

"Imagine something positive happening right now!" is a simple mental exercise that helps to make this shift of direction. It is a nice game to play and a useful technique for changing the direction of our thoughts. "Imagine that whatever is happening now is the very best beginning for the whole of the rest of my life!", is another.

When things are not going well, these exercises or games for the imagination will be harder than when life is rosy. They will sound like the stuff of wishful thinking. But they keep us receptive to the positive and open to opportunity, and facing in the right direction.

Our culture may have made a major error in emphasising, as it does today, bad news, violence and gloomy outlooks for us to feast upon. If we cannot change the culture, at least we can exercise our own minds to seek out more of the plus for ourselves. Humans are very responsive to the images they give themselves or receive from around them. When all the emphasis is negative, bodies, minds and spirits inevitably experience a big downward pull that affects more and more people in modern society. We surely need to keep creating better pictures and positive attitudes to use. When we recall stories of heroism that nations and individuals are proud of we are also strengthening our concepts of courage and generous actions as important qualities we all have and can share and use to make our human race special. Nowadays we tend to denigrate or undermine such behaviours or produce ulterior motives for them.

It is true that cruel and violent behaviours and ulteriot motives abound in our world. Human nature has some horrifying things in its history, and we have a genetic make up with a lot of negative patterns in it. Plenty of bad things have happened, still do, and will continue to happen. But plus and minus both exist, and the feasts that our imagination can best build upon for righting wrongs, solving problems and working towards cooperative and happy living are positive ones. To look at life more positively we should use our negatives only as a challenge to work to make things better, not as a continuous parade of the blame and criticism and disappointment and rift-making that are the stuff of today's more cynical media culture.

This does not mean that we should close eyes and ears to the world's horrors or ignore suffering and live in a fantasy world. We do need to explore what went wrong. We always have the task of trying to heal and overcome and sometimes even go to war with the minuses. But for a health bringing use of the imagination that can benefit ourselves and others we should learn to keep turning our attention towards the opportunities in front of us, even in cruel situations, and to positive solutions and positive visions. Great statesmen are usually doing this and inspire their people with their vision, but one sometimes suspects that journalists do their training in *blame, anger and criticism* schools.

Changing the emphasis from minus to plus in the mental world is closely parallel to turning our attention away from bodily compression and towards lengthening, opening up and three dimensional extension physically. We can use the physical example to illuminate those values in our mental lives. In a spiritual sense, too, the emphasis goes towards being the best human being we can manage to be ourselves and in relation to other people, rather than pillorying everyone else for their badness and for making a mess of our world.

We surely have an existential duty to use human consciousness in this positive direction, in the direction of opening up the human possibilities wherever we can, rather than closing them down and wallowing in "Ain't it awful!" The imagination is our ally here. Don't just use it for escape purposes. It is so good at using the images with which we feed it to create the reality around us that we should be glad to employ it positively. It is like choosing good food rather than bad when we look for bodily nourishment.

Be Very Plus About You

The crucial groundwork when exercising the imagination positively, is to start on our own self worth. (Go back to Chapter 1 if you feel this to be a selfish exercise.) If we are short of self value we may find it quite hard to be of much use to others. Gloomy pictures of and statements about our personal share of abilities, prospects, worth and fitness only undermine us and are very depressing for those we are with. They pull others down all around us too. We can break out of a habit of self negation if we keep checking what our mind is up to, and seeing that our inner judgements about ourselves and our capabilities and achievements stay full of confidence and bright and positive possibilities.

It is quite a challenge to exchange long-term feelings of inadequacy or old habits of self criticism for new and life-enhancing pictures about ourselves. Some people have more trouble with this than others. But it is worthwhile to take up this challenge and cultivate this skill because the more we grumble, the more life will surely hand us events to grumble about. Yet the more we appreciate life and our healthy place in it, the more treats and miracles do come along to be appreciated, and the more effectively we can make a positive difference in it ourselves.

There are many facets of this need for self value. Other people, for example, tend to judge us as we judge ourselves. As well as the things we say about ourselves, our body language and posture are always telling others how we feel about ourselves. One American charm school teaches its clients that they will never marry a millionaire if they have a slumped posture or apologetic attitudes! We may not want that particular motivation, but the story illustrates a truth about posture and self worth and the way both of these directly affect people we meet.

Affirmations and visualisations are both useful mental exercises if self esteem needs a boost. If marrying a millionaire seems a good idea to you, give your imagination free rein to paint pictures about that! But be sure to accompany that inner exercise with practical work to reinforce the changes you seek. Brilliant as the mind and imagination are, their work is only part of the whole enterprise for positive change.

The Effects are Not Imaginary

As discussed in outline in Chapter 1, there is scientific evidence that positive attitudes, created only in our minds, do affect us positively physically, and it is comforting to know that our hunches about this have a firm seal of approval from the scientific world. In laboratory experiments thoughts have been found to produce measurable changes in blood pressure, heart beat, skin temperature and pain thresholds.

The neurotransmitters, hormones and other chemicals of the nervous system are responding continuously to the thinking side of our experience and we can deliberately choose to use this fact well. A national newspaper quoted Neil Kinnock reflecting on a political misfortune, when he gave up his position as leader of the opposition in Parliament, saying: "Resentment is an extremely bitter diet, and eventually a poisonous one. I have no desire to make my own toxins". The body's reactions to our thoughts and imaginings are by no means imaginary and this fact is clearly recognised quite widely by practical politicians as well as psychologists and counsellors.

Less obviously than the health prospects, even the very circumstances of life seem to cheer up when our outlook is positive and our actions generous towards ourselves, others and life in general. This is harder to explain. There may not be scientific research about attitudes affecting circumstances, but there is plenty of day-to-day evidence that prosperity and happy relationships do seem to be correlated with a climate of positive attitudes and positive words and actions. We have also all seen misfortune and accidents, not just ill health, dogging the footsteps of angry and unhappy people. They may believe that the misfortunes came first and attitudes next, but sometimes we can see that it may be the other way round.

The full health of our body mind and spirit, and I suggest, our culture, needs abundantly positive images to sustain it in the midst of the negative pressures around us. It makes sense to take not only some thought but some positive exercise, too, in the direction of those images.

Anti-Gravity for Minds

Positive practices for minds produce a positive outward pressure right through the negatives about us, akin to the anti-gravity system our body has evolved to cope with the physical force of gravity. "Here is this strong downward pull, and here is my human ability to rise out of it". The *pressure* then becomes the force that *loads the springs* of our positive movement in this mental sense. "Here comes a challenge! Right! Here comes my best attempt at a wholly positive response to that".

Another plus image is that of the human being who can shine like the sun, right through any darkness and regardless of any clouds in our way!

A first visualisation exercise for the imagination is to upgrade the personal picture of your own fitness and see it as intrinsically a radiant expansive force of health flowing outwards from you in all directions! Like the proprioceptive system, it knows how to work against other pressures.

Don't think of your inner healing powers as an army of soldiers fighting desperately and defensively behind barricades against an invading armies of germs and disease. Imagine your body as sharing a universe benignly with many other evolved organisms but emitting such a powerful radiation of incandescently positive life itself, that the ones bringing disease just do not belong with you and can find no way in. They meet this outward radiation head on and realise they must leave quickly.

Once again, we may have to go *over the top* with our mind's images, just to break a habit of using thoughts, words, actions and imaginations too often and too absent-mindedly in their negative mode. If disease does appear, offer it courteous but short-term accommodation only and politely show it the best way to leave!

Visualisation in Training Programmes

Before trying these exercises, we should take a look first at the ways in which visualisations work. Basically any happy visualised images are stimulating the right side of the brain. In a sports or other training session the coach will be concentrating some of the training to this very creative region. He or she will keep the trainee's left brain happy by providing practical verbal instructions, but then will take the right brain right away on imaginative journeys towards better and better skills.

The trainee is then shown videos and films and given anecdotal examples or live demonstrations of other people's inspiring expert skills, and is asked to create sparklingly positive mental pictures for him or herself. S/he will settle down to visualise a better-than-ever high jump or ski-run, or sale or business performance, with a wonderful ease and a superbly successful outcome.

The coach knows that after enjoying an exciting fantasy trip into a new level of skill, unhampered by rules, criticisms or mistakes, the body/mind will work away behind the scenes towards making that experience come true. He knows, too, that streams of "No!"s or "Wrong!"s go deeply into the nervous system and hinder progress. He knows that every healthy organism has an intrinsic drive to live to the full and optimise its potential, and that each good picture and example inspires and feeds that inner drive.

Everyday Uses

We are using these psychological techniques intuitively in any case, even when we are not aware of them, whenever we simply admire a nice posture, a good game of tennis or a craftsman or window cleaner doing a good job. Admiration itself feeds positive pictures and ideas and possibilities into our minds. A little self admiration is not out of place either! As long as we carry a pleasing image of the suppleness and uprightness we want in our own life and our value as a human being too, our right brain will work subtly towards those images for us.

The Left Brain as Judge

As we noted in Chapter 1, the left brain does the mind's critical work. It does also have an annoying tendency to judge even our best efforts very harshly, and we need to accept that such critical alertness is part of its job. But we can keep it away from excessive negative preoccupation if we give it some useful tasks to do. If you have a habit of criticising yourself and others, it is your left brain that is the culprit. It has probably taken over the role of an authoritarian parent or teacher from the past, and we can start to see its habit of complaining in that light of replaying old tapes. For our own safety it believes it should keep us in a totally secure and stable situation, with other people very well behaved too, with firm rules all round and not too many risks.

A practical technique for disarming this watchful and anxious left brain judge, is to count how many times you criticise yourself or other people in one whole day! That will give it something interesting to do. But in doing that exercise it will also get a subtle glimpse into its own workings and will notice how automatic it has become. Fortunately, the left brain is clever enough to learn quite quickly from such an exercise and after a few such experiments will begin to moderate its habit of producing a stream of criticisms.

It is not helpful to criticise even our own left brain for being critical! Harsh judging of any kind, as we see in human arguments, only leads to a defensive strengthening up of that which is being judged. If we are sympathetic to its activities it will relax its belligerence and be willing to change and help us in very positive ways. We need to give our left brain the safe and secure feeling such as a counsellor or doctor provides in a therapeutic and healing relationship, or a parent looking after the development of a child.

Love and support are appropriate in our relationship to any part of the brain as to any part of our family, our society or institutions or even the press, if we want it to make positive changes and really do its best. It may seem bizarre to treat our brain as we treat friends or to treat friends as we treat our brain, but the idea is a practical one. Support and acknowledgement are good for us all in every situation.

The Right Brain – mini-exercises

Another simple warm-up exercise for stimulating the visual imagination is to relax any tension first and then devote a few minutes solely to visualising some of the positive qualities we want to increase in our lives. Close your eyes and look inwardly at some specific areas in your own life, not just fitness matters, and see them getting better. This is not an idle activity if we use it well. It is not the same as day dreaming. We are helping to make our wants clearer and more explicit to ourselves. We can then shift back from this little right brain excursion to the practicality of finding ways of making these nice things come true. We can have our own imaginary support team if we like, gods and goddesses, gurus and angels, and our own secret place to go to mentally when doing this visualisation.

For a direct right brain mental boost for physical fitness, try closing your eyes and imagining a favourite scene with you physically happy and active in it. You are moving gracefully, alone or with friends, playing, swimming, running, perhaps sailing, skiing or flying, with easy, uninhibited and graceful movement. This right brain game is stimulating for vision as well as liberating for joints and muscles. On a country walk, be a squirrel in the trees, leaping from branch to branch, or a bird soaring in the sky.

Before a journey, always visualise arriving safely. Don't dwell on possible hazards and discomforts. Believe it or not, you will have far fewer problems and a much happier ride. If emergencies do arise, you will be so relaxed and confident you will easily cope with them and be able to help other people, too.

The Visualisation Exercise

This longer exercise is a good way of using the mind and imagination to bring extra harmony and efficiency to the mind's own way of operating. It requires a small step of detachment to do this, and this is a useful exercise in itself. The mind spends a lot of its time operating on automatic pilot, but while we are in the process of observing and exercising it we can introduce new ideas and a little supervision and guidance.

We divide the brain into four main volumes for this exercise, not just the two halves already discussed. There are no such rigid areas, of course. In fact, we probably have many more than four different ways of managing our mental challenges, with much overlapping of function, and they are not housed in totally water tight compartments. But in this way we can observe some clashes of interest and some differing approaches and priorities operating.

It does not even matter if your tongue is in your cheek while you do this exercise. Even if you only ever do it once, it can bring a vivid new awareness of the possibilities within you of *getting it all together*.

Imagine four main volumes of the brain:

❒ On the left: See all your logic, verbal and *one-at-a-time* skills operating from the left side

❒ On the right: Your visual and creative skills, with integrative, *all-at-once* abilities and insights

❒ In the fore brain: All your forward looking vision and planning ahead

❒ In the hind brain: Tenacious loyalty, holding on to safe and well established habits. Expert survival skills from a long genetic and cultural inheritance.

Lie or sit comfortably, eyes closed. Let go of unwanted tensions everywhere and start to get in touch with this hidden management team in your brain.

Linking left and right

Spread your hands along the sides of the head and imagine you are enclosing one whole hemisphere under each hand. Pause like this. You may even get the feeling that one side is bigger or perhaps just a little dominant in the left/right partnership.

Now talk to these two sides of your brain in imagination, in turn. Use your own words, and be friendly and at home with them. If you feel embarrassed talking to your brain, think of the tough footballers and practical businessmen who have found new successes through very various positive mental visualisations.

Thank your left brain first, though it does not matter where you start. Thank it for its great work in managing all your verbal skills and time tables and logic and so forth. Let it know that you think it quite brilliant and really appreciate all that it does for you.

Then thank your right brain, cupped under the right hand, for the brilliant ideas it has, and the way it edges you into creative activities big or small, like business projects or research plans or making birthday cards or music or a new look in clothes. Tell it that you love its special talents and all that it does to brighten life for you and everyone you know.

Then invite these two sides to bring their differing qualities into a little closer harmony. Ask them to cultivate their friendship more actively. Invite them to cooperate and trust each other and use each other's skills and expertise. Tell them that life lets us make a successful outcome even from a big diversity of talents and beliefs and even entrenched biases if we negotiate together rather than fighting each other.

Play a manager's role. Point out some of the obvious ways in which these two rather different departments can now help and support each other more actively. The left side can help the right to be more practical, and the right side can encourage the left to be a little less stuffy and judgmental and a lot more playful. You know best where you could use such cooperation between the fanciful creativity that your right brain undoubtedly has, and the logical, but perhaps overly cautious good sense over on the left side.

Linking front and back

Change the hand positions next and talk to the front and back of the brain together. Use one hand to hold the upper forehead this time, and the other to reach to the back of your head, almost into the upper spine. The primitive and protective hind-brain developed long ago from the spinal nervous system and is right back on the spinal stem.

Treat the frontal area as the one that is entirely *up front* and looking towards the future with optimism. See it as creating new visions and setting the goals for your life. I call this the Dick Whittington department! When we make a really firm commitment here, all the other departments take their cue from it. We intuitively start doing whatever needs to be done next, like walking to London, in Dick Whittington's case. For us this might mean getting organised for our sports or exercise programme, packing for a holiday, telephoning the plumber or measuring up for new curtains. When the commitment is real and strong, all the other steps fall into place, one by one.

The bigger fore brain is one of the more recent acquisitions that make us distinctively human. When you look towards the big vistas of the future with it in this way, don't analyse the risks and details at first. Just see the goal or the results you want very clearly and strengthen your commitment to them. Offer plenty of love and admiration and encouragement to this adventurous part of the brain that works towards your positive visions of the future.

As the hind brain is much older in evolutionary terms it is still tied into all the primitive and basic qualities that life needed in the past and still needs, of course, like safety and survival. It is very, very good at them. Sometimes too good! Its analysis of risk, for example, can often be a little too cautious.

The hind brain is also managing many basic automatic functions on which your body relies, like removing your hand from a hot stove before you have time to apply logic to the situation, or turning to run from danger, real or sometimes only imagined, very fast. It desperately wants you to survive, so it employs strong imperatives to be absolutely sure you do.

Talk to these rather oppositely motivated departments as you did to left and right, separately first, with friendly thanks. See yourself as a benevolent manager and ask for more cooperation between them. The hind brain needs to be handled especially tenderly, as you would a child. She is intelligent and devotedly on your side, but often tries to hold you back.

Nevertheless, this strong team member is quite capable of appreciating your up-to-date interests and commitments. With your encouragement and guidance she can learn to distinguish between real emergencies and situations that seem frightening only because they are unknown and she will like to cooperate. Thank her for all that fantastic strength and amazing loyalty and offer her your love and appreciation and trust.

As you put these two in touch and encourage a cooperation between them, point out to the fore brain how wise the hind brain really is. Explain that it is in her nature to be protective and that you know she is anxious sometimes, but her advice is often very sound.

By making friendly links between all the quadrants you have visited you will be balancing their differing contributions. They need each other and they make a great team. As team leader you are making an introduction that may never have been made before, and may only need to be made this once. A new relationship and new cooperation can now begin. Each department or facet of your thinking can become more open to feedback from the others.

And that is all! It does not have to be serious and you don't have to believe that you have four people in your head! Just enjoy using the inventiveness of your imagination to promote a positive new partnership in your mental functioning. We can initiate at least an awareness of a possibility for greater mental flexibility and harmony in our own mental functioning.

After this exercise, as with the body work, always relax for a few moments while its messages are taken on board. These need time to filter through the various interfaces to enter the organism as a whole, not just to the part you worked with. Then go straight to whatever tasks present themselves, knowing that you have a more balanced and much stronger inner team supporting everything you do.

Affirmation Exercises

I have some reservations about affirmations where they are simply the recitation of words. It is true that with much repetition the ideas embodied in any verbal statements about ourselves will find their way into our subconscious mind and can make changes for good or bad in our attitudes and effectiveness. But as our verbal and intellectual side can sometimes operate with a lot of cynicism and suspicion, so I stress the need to use both sides of the brain at once, with pictures as well as words.

If you can picture the positive results you are looking for at the same time as affirming that new reality verbally, perhaps writing it as well as speaking it, then the left/right team will be much more powerful in their double harness. We are much more likely to succeed when we can *see* ourselves taking on a new job, for example, rather than when we *can't imagine* ourselves in that role.

A words-only affirmation can also make us feel dishonest and this undermines our self worth and might cancel out any benefit. Our use of language is very much a part of the way in which we are true to ourselves and true to others. It can feel all wrong to be stating: "I feel wonderful!", if you don't. A minor change of expression can help us past this problem. "I feel fine!" allows scope for further improvement while still speaking of a dawning positive state.

An inner visualisation of a desired result like a brilliant tennis performance, seems a more private exercise and can feel quite respectable. We can legitimately make a playfully realistic inner picture of ourselves in a quite different state. Creating words and pictures together is like an extension of that right brain picture making exercise, but including language.

Approach the technique of affirmations gently if they seem to be cheating, because our personal integrity is very important. Coax the suspicious left brain. Tell it you are conducting a private experiment and ask it to assess the results. Then take a very small positive statement about yourself. Try: "I am already a wee bit further on the way to the much better fitness I want, and I believe these exercises are beginning to make a small but positive difference". Although cautious, this is definitely plus. It is heading in the right direction. It is the beginning of a turn around and if you had a lot of momentum in the opposite direction of pessimism, then like turning a big ocean liner, it has to be tackled quite slowly.

Eventually your choice of words will work much better for you than mine, because they match your unique needs and visions. My examples below are really for priming the pump of your own creative ideas. You know best which areas of your life you want to affirm and strengthen. Take these as examples to practise with and then find better ones.

Relax comfortably and well aligned, either standing, sitting or lying, and take a few moments to release muscle tension consciously.

Close your eyes but inwardly look ahead as if at the new imagined reality. See In your imagination the results you want as you put them clearly into words, inwardly, aloud or in writing. It may be difficult to do both at the same time, especially if you are writing your affirmations. In that case alternate inner pictures with inner words. State or write your affirmation and at once see its results in a lively and positive picture. Repeat each one several times, taking time with each repetition to see as well as to hear them.

Always use the first person and the present tense for affirmations. If we put our fitness affirmations in a vague or a future mode, like hopes, they tend to stay vague and unrealised! "I will be slimmer tomorrow" will almost certainly retreat indefinitely.

Choose one of the following to experiment with but then make positive affirmations and create inner pictures that are all your own.

"I am naturally supple and fit and healthy".

"I am naturally active, energetic and enthusiastic".

"I am expert at shedding excess tensions whether active or still".

"I heal quickly now from illness and all hurts, whether bodily or emotional".

"I shed resentments and anxieties quickly".

"I love and appreciate myself and all others".

"I am naturally happy, loving, generous and wise".

"I encourage the two sides of my brain to work together. Their cooperation is a flourishing reality in my life and work".

"I am very skilful at discovering a positive opportunity where things have seemed to be bleak".

Remember to acknowledge in any case, with a positive verbal affirmation that you are a fine person and fully worthy of a place in the universal scheme of things! "I have a valuable place in the world", "I love and approve of myself", or "I feel good about myself," are fundamental to our satisfying participation in life, and to our contribution to others and to our health.

As with visualisations and all the other affirmations they need the backing of your willingness and commitment to work in that direction too. To stress this practical aspect, and escape from the trap of mere wishful thinking, then add to each and every one, as you make it, "and I am exercising regularly in that area to make sure that I keep these qualities always alive".

EXERCISE SECTION 12

Can We Exercise the Human Spirit?

The Exercises

Introducing the S-Factor

Spirit is a big abstract word and there are no limits set as human beings try to define it. Whether we have one or not, or are one or part of a bigger one, and can or cannot summon or consult spirit, are questions with many answers. But if we live as if we have one the concept will be real to us. Look in the dictionary and you find many interpretations. Read poetry or literature, and references to spirit cover a huge field. Follow a particular religion or study an oriental philosophy and the concept widens and widens.

When I talk about a human spirit in this book of practical exercises, it is with the sense of opening ourselves up to its beneficent presence and its mysterious flow, not pinning it down to specific properties or behaviours. If we see our own share of human spirit as an entirely positive something that flows within us for good, and also crosses all gaps between us and other people for mutual good, we have plenty to work on in an everyday way. We can find things to do to open us up to such a big positive force. We can bring it into an exercise scheme.

Some human activities seem to shut out all spiritual involvement. Other activities, thoughts or words do encourage it to flow more freely. This, then, is our area for exercise. It will be in activities that refresh our own spirit and also link us with other people. It is a very wide field but I have chosen the very natural and practical area of giving and receiving and especially of giving. There are easy parallels here with the life-giving extension and outwardness on which bodies thrive.

So why does this chapter not simply say: "Do good to others, it is good for you too!", and leave it at that? Once again the intention of this introduction is largely to provoke thought and expand awareness, awareness being a major tool for transformation or positive change.

The exercises are ones that work for US, this time, not for you and me separately. I am neither a philosopher nor a spiritual expert. But this exploration around human generosity may stimulate your own enquiry, and then, even if my picture is inadequate, you can use it to sharpen your own and range much further in what spirit means to you.

From Minus to Plus for Spirits

I have chosen a positive definition. We traditionally have had both angels and devils in our spiritual imagery and may be scared of the bad ones. But if you have too many evil spirits in your philosophy, please leave them behind at this point. They probably don't exist! They certainly do not need exercising! Use your imagination positively and recruit as many *good angels* as you would like to support you.

In preparation, close your eyes and mentally consign all the negatives of the past, of every variety, to an imaginary universal reservoir, dustbin or black hole, and say goodbye to them. Sweep them away! Like the unwanted negatives of physical and emotional tensions, we have often held on to them unnecessarily and they have held us back. And as before, the exercises we do actively will help this process of ushering the *baddies* out of our lives.

Turning then to the plus, we will explore some of the abstract spiritual positives such as good will, appreciation, love, forgiveness, blessings and many varieties of human generosity that work between human beings even without physical actions or words. We can find simple exercises to take us across gaps between people at all levels, in consciously positive thoughts, consciously positive words, and consciously positive deeds.

Why should I?

Knowing that these exercises are going to be mostly about positive interpersonal behaviour we might well want to hold back. "Why me? Why not the state, my boss or my spouse or family? What I would really like is for someone else to be doing all of that generosity and goodwill in my direction, towards and for me! I don't see why I should do any of them! It sounds rather like hard work!"

We may even feel we have a right to be at the receiving end of everyone else's, the state's and the universe's generosity and we probably add a few grumbles about our rights and about the world owing us a living. There is, unfortunately, quite a big emphasis in human nature and certainly in our culture on trying to race our neighbour to a larger slice of the cake, so to speak, rather than looking for ways to contribute to him or her.

In formulating a citizen's charter, patient's charter or consumer's charter, for example, even the government's emphasis has often been on the goodies we are entitled to receive rather than any responsibility to earn such largesse or give anything back to society ourselves. We may even have some genetic instructions about this bias towards taking, because individuals are programmed to survive and when survival is at stake we are still likely to take the me-first imperative automatically.

Western culture, in particular, has prized competition for a long time and much of our commercial life has a strong bias towards personal gain. We quite often treat the suppliers of our wants and needs rather unfairly, imagining that our needs are paramount. But aware human spirits can do better than this. Our survival is not at stake. We need not always cheat a little for a business advantage, trample on others to score a point or exploit a creative talent or a vulnerable person. Humans have the opportunity to do better than grab automatically if they will stop to think. Our spirit actually loves to contribute to others.

Another important fact about good deeds is that we cannot force anyone else to do them. So if we want any of the desirable top-down, *spiritual* extras to be happening anywhere, we have an adult responsibility to do some of them. It is this outward and creative expansive directedness, now at a spiritual level, that probably needs more conscious exercise than the claiming and demanding side.

We obviously cannot personally supply all the needs of the universe single handed! And it is wonderful to enjoy receiving bounty from all around us, too. But our only certainty about life's abstract, good, contributing qualities is that while we are producing them, even in our own smallest positive actions, their existence is guaranteed. (I know that we are all doing this in any case, by the way, but this exploration is still about increasing our awareness in this matter.).

The Tai Chi recommendation for practising any of its exercises and forms, solo or interpersonally, says rather facetiously: "If you feel like practising, practise. If you don't feel like practising, practise." This is a good rule for generating any of our best behaviours of spirit too. Such exercise is not hard work. It is not a chore. It is not even a moral requirement. It is a positive gift of health for ourselves as well as for any recipient of our goodwill.

Tonics or Warm-ups for Spirits

Physically

All the right-brain-friendly activities that we intuitively feel are good for our spirits can be used for warming up or opening up. Use these often to give your whole B/M/S a treat. Take a walk in the garden or countryside. Play with children. Look at works of art you love or read literature that inspires you to value the good in human nature.

Relaxed bodily actions such as yawning, laughing, singing, cross-crawl, stretching or just swinging the arms or legs as children do, all help to wake up and invigorate the whole B/M/S organism. Opening up physically in length and width, and mentally into alertness, both enlarge a doorway for the spirit. Openness of spirit is reflected in openness of body and mind. Someone has said that minds, like parachutes, work better open than closed, which is a nice way of remembering the life-giving opportunity of the quality of total openness for bodies too.

Opening up physically also acts expressively as a body language. It is welcoming to others so it backs up the spirit in helping us across the gaps that might seem to separate people. Even on the telephone, your communication will be more fully expressed and received if you open up and lengthen physically, three dimensionally while you talk. We are more present to others as well as to ourselves when we respect our bodily integrity.

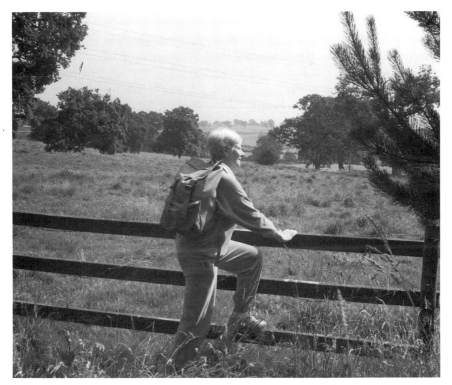

Taking a walk in the countryside is a tonic for the spirit

Mentally

All generous thoughts as well as positive verbal expressions are spiritually energising. We can use them very simply yet very awarely. Try "I feel good!" "This will be great!" Such mental warm-ups are colloquially called *psyching up*. The mind is getting the whole organism ready to contribute positively. Eventually we hardly need to psych up. A well exercised spirit is vitality itself and is always ready to take spontaneous positive action.

Socially

It is liberating to share some of our positive outward going activities, especially with other plus spirits. Friends who are cheerfully positive reinforce us in our own plusness and help us to feel the uselessness of some of our negative attitudes. Their vitality inspires our own spirit directly. We go away from their company enriched, ready to share that same gift with someone else.

Warming up with appreciation

Appreciation works to expand us. There is a positive spiritual thrust going on when we outwardly express our appreciation of things and actions that we see as good. It is good for our spirit and a first-class skill to cultivate and exercise. We can expand our awareness of the way the whole human enterprise holds together and works when we appreciate more of it. We open up more pathways across it and the whole network becomes more interesting.

There is a positive power in appreciation that releases body/mind tensions miraculously, and it can work wonders for people around us too. We can warm up by exercising our appreciation at any time, verbally or as a silent, inner recognition, for real spiritual benefit and a little general health tonic.

Be warmly, openly and straightforwardly thankful for everything you enjoy! Glow with appreciation, whether towards the sun for its warmth or the trees for their shade. Become more aware of the many ways in which life is enriched. Forget for a while the flood of rivalries and disasters and ill feelings. Appreciate parents, children, family and friends for loving you, even if you have doubts sometimes. Appreciate your neighbours for inviting you in, for gossiping over the fence or sharing their holiday snaps with you.

Appreciate doctors and dentists for their care, farmers, market gardeners, tea growers, food and wine producers and distributors, too, for making all these things available. Keep going! Appreciate the foods and drinks themselves, and the bountiful earth. Appreciate even things you may take for granted or want to criticise such as the railway system, politicians, tax men and supermarkets. However fallible or annoying they sometimes seem, they are doing very valuable work. Use appreciation as a field or climate in which your spirit thrives.

The lazier opposites of appreciation are blaming and complaining. (The very words sound depressing!) Complaining, or whinging, is often only an automatic habit pattern, an unthinking flow of *minus-speak*, welling up from past grudges. But if we drift into it we are likely to become almost addicted to it and keep whining more and more.

Our culture seems to encourage us to complain and it is very easy to feel superior when we do it! But a complaint is only valuable when it is directed straight to the one complained about. It is too easy to find fault everywhere and to give ourselves a quite poisonous diet of these negatives. Indignation and anger usually accompany complaining and they are far from beneficial to bodies or minds or to effective problem solving. They are rarely necessary even when there is much to be done and we are impatient and wishing that everything was perfect.

The critical faculty has both a positive and a negative side. We need something equivalent to our anti-gravity system here, a little positive thrust, to let us escape the lure of its downward pressures. Exercising appreciation gives us very useful practice of its constructive and positive mode! There is so much that is good around us it should not be difficult to find ways to practise this one if we keep our minds and eyes open for it.

Try at least 10 deliberate statements of modest but definite appreciation every day! "This tastes good" at breakfast or "Lovely day!" when we meet a fellow human being. Add a smile to cross the gap as well. Each of these small utterances can be seen as making a positive spiritual contribution. They are gifts.

We have all been practising these life enhancing things for years, of course, without thinking about them, but it does not spoil them to bring them into positive awareness. Acknowledge the action of spirit here and they become part of the maintenance of a rich holistic awareness in our life.

Exercises that Work for Spirits

The main exercises for the S member of the B/M/S team are about exercising love, forgiveness, and giving and blessing, all of which bring important health benefits. We need not be sentimental about these activities. If we are to *cultivate* our spirit, these all give us exercise in a faculty that easily extends us beyond ourselves. They are activities we associate with God, gods or guardian angels and we may have been taught to feel pious about them, yet we know that human beings are also able to practise them. While the body/mind exercises are all solo and domestic, these outward extended practices can link us straightforwardly with other spirits and work as widely as we care to take them.

To probe into these four a little, we can look at love first in its evolutionary setting where it began in the world of time, space and biology. In our species it then takes a higher meaning as human consciousness enters the evolutionary scene and we accept spirit as well as body/mind.

Consciousness is also a product of evolution, of course. Nothing we do can be separate from the natural world and in her own way, Nature is probably observing closely, to see if consciousness has any long-term advantages over its classic, pre-thought method of survival of the fittest. If the consciousness experiment should fail, she will carry on with the basic evolutionary processes without us and new situations will bring some new experiments.

Exercising Love

All animals that care for their young have those biological beginnings tightly programmed into their lives. So do we. Love has worked for survival. But we can think of the maturing possibility for love as if it has two directions: the biologically driven variety and the more spiritual and we operate in both. I call the evolved, programmed, *Darwinian* mode its *bottom-up* direction, derived totally from the genetic patterning. And then our *top-down* spiritual direction applies to the higher human values we have created for love as our species has matured. As children of both these systems, we can exercise love in both these ways.

Love changes the direction of its emphasis as we grow older. We mature biologically and we grow in awareness of humanity around us. As mature adults we become more and more willing to give love, as well as still enjoying receiving it, and in most people this is a natural progression.

In terms of higher human values this directional shift is also a progression. We may express the higher qualities of love as *God-given*, to try to explain the mystery of its higher status. Whether it derives from a spirit as infinite and infinitely good as thought can take us, or from a summing up or distillation of human values, our best way with love is to do it. We can clearly see each individual life adding its own small quota of spiritual love and strengthening those higher values in the way it lives and operates among other people.

Our first experience of love was in the bottom-up pattern, in the biological bond with our parents. It all seemed to come in one direction then, our way. So we may tend to expect for a long time that that is the right and proper direction for love. There were no conditions then. All we had to do was to snuggle into our mother's breast. If we cried for more attention it usually came.

But infants meet shock after shock as they grow up. There are always other people in the mother's life and other interests, needs and responsibilities. Sometimes a temporary withdrawal of parental care would have felt like abandonment for ever. Part of a parent's job is to prepare the child to be self reliant and able to cope with problems and social living, but the shocks along the way will often feel, to the small child, like disaster or tragedy.

Infants are instinctively wonderfully loving too, of course. They love to give and share and they gaze with rapture at the mother who loves them. But their early expectation is that they are omnipotent and permanently central where love is concerned. Eventually they have to yield to the realities of relating to more and more people and not always being central even in their mother's life. The bigger complex arenas of family life, school, friendships and community open up and widen out.

That whole experience of increasing separation is an existential one. It happens to each individual inevitably as it struggles from infancy to maturity. But although universal, each individual experience is very real, often acutely painful, always unique, and often leaves scars.

When we first faced that apparent competition for love, we experimented with ways of getting our share of attention! Sometimes we sulked. Sometimes we tried dramatic temper tantrums or extra charm. If very frightened we might have withdrawn inside and pulled the shutters down. Between infancy and adulthood we probably tried everything, and it would be natural to hold on to the behaviour patterns that seemed to work for us.

We call this process of adaptation our *conditioning*. And most of these acquired patterns relate to the small child needing to know it is loved.

It is no wonder that in the tough processes of learning to adapt socially we acquire muscle imbalance, mental rigidities and many varieties of emotional crippling unless we are very, very lucky. Our attitudes began to take shape in that process, and the word attitude is very close in meaning to the word posture. Body and mind were in it together and responded in closely similar ways.

In the next chapter we look at ways in which we can take a second look at some of the emotional tensions that could have originated in early years and then stay trapped and dominant. It may be possible to let go of some of these, little by little. If we can, the health benefits are enormous and all our relationships can become warmer and more openly loving.

Those are the biological, bottom-up origins of love. Growing up in and then out of that process, we have then built up such a strong picture of the value of loving and caring that we value these for themselves and not just for their survival value. Love, along with awareness has become special to our species and we increasingly value being suppliers as well as receivers of love.

A proper love of self is also plus

Part of our physical and mental well-being lies in the necessity to be a healthy producer of love for ourselves, too! The rest of the world may be too busy to give us all that we would like. There may be other priorities about.

If we cannot love ourselves, our love for other people will suffer. We seem to have only one quality or climate of love to give, and the same quality that brings health to our own life flows also between us and others. If we hate ourselves, some of that hate leaks out and we begrudge love to other people. There is an inner security when we do love ourselves wholesomely, that makes its presence felt in all our relationships. It is a very nice human duty to put ourselves high on any list of people we love, and then go on extending that list. Do put it into your fitness programme and your first aid cabinet.

At times we should be right at the top of our own list and give ourselves some special personal treats. And we should always find time for basic self caring, including exercising well and providing our body and mind with good nourishment. It is essential to full health to feel really good about oneself and to feel happy about all that which we are, say and do. A first exercise in love is to practise loving ourselves right through our mistakes and failures and omissions as well, as we might love a very good friend. This is only selfish if self is the only person we honour in this way.

There is no need for any detailed instructions for exercising love. Warm up by doing something nice for yourself today and every day, openly and without apology, and continue by doing something nice for someone else, too. Let those you love know that you do indeed love them. Recognise the spiritual value of love in all its forms, even if we bungle it sometimes. And use the physical images of health, extension and the anti-gravity possibilities of the whole human organism to build up a more loving world in the top-down sense. Love is no longer just for lovers, mothers and babies.

The Forgiveness Exercise

Forgiveness is another spiritual bonus and it, too, releases tensions all round. Like love it has acquired some overtones of sentimentality and could benefit from shedding these. If you are wondering what on earth it has to do with fitness, well, it works right in the body's chemistry for good, and in the muscles to release trapped tightnesses, and it works *out there* in all our relationships to broaden and strengthen them. It is undoubtedly good for us and should be exercised.

The word forgiveness sounds smug and it takes a little care to avoid the pitfall of smugness. It is only an illusion that any forgiver is ever superior to the person forgiven. No one is superior or inferior in the human network. We are each *top* in any case. We should feel glad about our shared human worth, and acknowledge the mixed goodness and badness in all of us, and truly forgive all those we have ever felt sore about, as one long on-going exercise.

Forgiveness, at its practical and spiritual best can be a sort of super-acceptance of people exactly as they are – sharing a planet, struggling to do their best, sometimes blind or driven, often making mistakes in a fast changing and ever challenging world. It is a completer of unfinished business and a bringer of health.

Again, it is a *climate* to live in, and one that must also include oneself, for we are also members of the human race. And it may need our conscious, top-down effort to sustain it, powered from a higher than biological sense. We probably have to remind ourselves that it is just as natural for people to be bad as to be good, and especially to notice that we are often bad ourselves and to accept those truths. Forgiving is doubly beneficial, of course, but probably most of its benefits come to the person who does it. Sometimes the person forgiven may not even notice, or may even have died, while the forgiver can be shedding quite a heavy load.

Self forgiveness, like the self respect of love, is powerful too. When we forgive our own shortcomings we also shed a weighty personal burden. Restrictive physical tensions can suddenly evaporate as guilt leaves us. We also grow more sympathetic to other people in all their mistakes and transgressions when we have forgiven ourselves for our own. As part of exercising love for yourself, forgive yourself for all the mistakes, *faux pas* and misdeeds for which you may have berated yourself in the whole of your life, however embarrassed or ashamed you have felt about them. Make a list and then burn it as you let them all go.

The past is neutralising itself in any case, and when we forgive past events it is like joining in with that neutralising process, accepting them as completely over, as nature herself accepts them. With forgiveness we clear the decks for increasing the supply and flow of love and health and healing and prospering.

The gods, gurus and guardian angels of our culture, religion or even of our personal imagination if we have no specific faith or religious experience, will bring a lot of support in this forgiveness enterprise. Since they accept and love us exactly as we are and forgive us unconditionally, they set us a wonderful example.

I like to expand the concept of forgiveness sometimes by forgiving a whole string of things one after another! If an infant spills milk, for example, once I have recovered my serenity, I deliberately forgive not just this infant for the mess, but all infants for being infants! I forgive infancy itself for being a part of growth. I forgive myself for being often quite infantile in my reactions. I forgive the evolutionary process for not leaping straight from the infancy of its single cell origins to a paradise of perfect beings who never ever spill milk! After such a wide ranging exercise, next time the reaction of annoyance can last a shorter time and acceptance and the job of clearing up will start sooner.

We can forgive the past and we can forgive and look more kindly towards the future, and we can forgive the flaws in our bodies and minds, our judgements or appetites, our history and our genes, as well as in our culture, other people and the whole world. Play this forgiveness game sometimes in a huge way. Spend a little exercise time on it. Forgive the *riddle of the universe* for being so fathomless, the human condition for not having all the answers and life for not going your way all the time. And then appreciate, love and forgive yourself for whatever experimental approach you and the human race have to use in living within this mystery.

If you believe that too much forgiveness or acceptance or appreciation or even love, could be a soppy mistake and might make us all too careless and easy going, ask yourself how much you would like to be forgiven for your own mistakes and appreciated just as you are. I guess it would number at least the *seventy times seven* of Jesus Christ's recommendation. Ask yourself, too, if there are any tightened parts of your anatomy that could perhaps be associated with some life-long grudges, guilts or hates, and start letting those tensions go, too. Then do several forgiveness exercises each day, however small.

Forgiving oneself is not the same as making excuses! We still need to make reparation and urge others to do the same when we or they have done real harm, and we may even sometimes need to fight for ourselves or someone else. But forgiveness heals and should be a part of picking ourselves up after mistakes or battles, facing in the plus direction again and getting on with the positive, more life-giving and health bringing side of life.

The Give/Receive Exercise

Giving is a good basic exercise for spirits.Don't think of it as do-gooding. It has an outwardness that, as for bodies and minds, brings release of tensions all round and enlivening energy to the whole organism. It is a fundamental plus for holistic fitness, it is easy to do, ranges widely, and operates at many levels. As making humanity work is a living and expanding process, so the outwardness of giving may need to have just a slight edge over the inwardness of receiving, in the network of relationships. A network in which taking and receiving were always given priority and no giving happened, would surely collapse inwards.

Gratitude, or receiving warmly, is the other half of the give/receive process. Done in a positive spirit it is also quite vital and expansive, and similarly frees tensions and brings health and energy. Speak/listen, buy/sell, produce/consume are similarly balanced communication dualities. They look like separate activities, but they work always together from two directions at once. And each side of each of these joint processes, if we look at it in this way, can be seen as a gift. From either side of these dual activities we contribute to each other and to our shared and individual health.

It was Jane Austen who noted that gratitude does not seem to come automatically, whereas the expectation of gratitude does! Yes! We do rather expect people to be grateful when we are the giver, but again that very fact alerts us to a balancing obligation to receive gifts in a positive way ourselves when they come our way. Giving one's gratitude can be a consciously positive and decidedly generous action, oiling the joints of the human structure, bringing the spiritual equivalents of synovial fluids and oxygen to lubricate and nourish the social skeleton.

Generosity is so multi-faceted and multi-levelled that again we need to explore our way around it if we want to exercise it more awarely. A tidying up job is a gift, either to oneself if it is at the back of a cupboard, or also to all who share our life if it is in a living room, work space or the street.

If you are a generous talker, be a generous listener, too. If a generous giver, be a generous receiver as well. Don't try to do both sides of any of these dualities at once. Value each side and give full value with it and enjoy taking turns. Listen all the time you are listening. Receive all the time you are receiving.

I was once at a party at which one of the guests entertained us throughout the meal with the full details, course by course, of a much more splendid banquet she had recently enjoyed somewhere else. It seemed quite hard to see our hostesses' own offerings overlooked. I learned from that experience that when I am a guest it is better to be fully at my hostess's party, receiving and enjoying, and to tell of its pleasures afterwards only in non-dinner-party situations. Tact is also an act of generosity.

In none of these dualities of give/receive is one side more good or more generous than the other. The one who learns contributes his interest and learning while the teacher gives his teaching. In some societies students formally thank the teacher at the end of a lesson. In martial arts classes this respect is an important part of the discipline. Sometimes after a lecture a speaker will thank the audience for being receptive. The giving and taking actions of these dual processes can both be performed with generosity.

Don't worry about being *conned* or seeming inappropriate sometimes when you give, just do it. A past snub can make us feel rejected and we can get into a habit of shrinking and, perhaps, even giving up giving which is definitely bad for us! Giving matters as a primary outwardness and it matters to our individual as well as our shared well-being. If your gift is not well received, shrug off the disappointment because you are still a giver. Your own spirit and your own self worth are healthy and alive when you give, at any level, even if you make mistakes, and whether your gift is well received or not.

Giving, like any other exercise, is not a full time occupation, of course. If giving becomes a preoccupation we should be looking at our motivation. We should balance our many ways of giving. By balancing, I do not mean by weighing and measuring! We do not always have to say "Yes", to every request, or pay back every kindness. "No thank you!" may often be an appropriate response. There can be times, too, when we are unable to give, or wish to interrupt a pattern of giving that has become stale or habit ridden. But we can awaken a positive awareness of a living balance in human intercourse, like muscle balance around a healthy body, when we see all this giving and receiving going on.

With awareness gained from physical injuries, we can learn not to feel hurt if someone does tread on our toes or does not give as much to us as we would like. And we can notice how creatively each small act of giving and receiving is playing its part in keeping the bigger human social organism healthy. We can appreciate that generosity in thought, word and deed helps to keep humanity human. And we can exercise our own more awarely. We can loosen up and stretch with small or large exercises in giving, and then we leave that practise time behind and let the benefits of its lessons just filter in.

Examples are hardly necessary. We know that we have millions of opportunities to contribute something in thought, word or deed to somebody else, friend or stranger. Ten contributions a day? Ten gifts of our listening? One of a letter or invitation? Some thankyous for generosity received or qualities appreciated? We need not set limits! If life ever starts to seem dull and boring or out of sorts, just check around to see if you have remembered the flow of healing generosity that belongs in vital human experience and tackle just one small exercise as a tonic.

I know perfectly well that we are all doing this and all the other spiritual exercises in any case, and we all deserve a pat on the back! Introducing them as exercises just brings the human spirit more awarely into the fitness scene. If we have lost some of its naturalness either in habits of tight-fistedness, or of an excessive self righteousness or even a fear about giving, a few exercises will bring the concept back more healthily into our lives. Dare I say that hand and facial and other bodily tensions may sometimes be released too? Make your own experiments. Your observant and clever left brain will draw its conclusions and act on them afterwards.

The Blessing Exercise

When we give someone our blessing, that seemingly minimal gift works for us, too. We can do it mentally or very quietly, but an open verbal expression gets across the gap more effectively between blesser and blessee. It is an action, usually a speech-action, akin to appreciation. Again it requires recognition of our equal worth with other human beings first, as it may seem a rather smug or arrogant thing to do. ("Who am I to be handing out blessings!").

Blessings are special to humans and to the spiritual support team of saints, gurus, gods and goddesses that our experience or imagination provide for us. Animals don't bless each other and we did not acquire this possibility from the bottom-up route of our animal inheritance. It is definitely a top-down activity. Machines cannot do it and it puts no strain on our mechanics!

But although so special and rather mysterious, it is also an everyday do-it-yourself healing action. Muscles relax, breathing expands, vision brightens, cheeks glow and our inner chemistry perks up as we wish happiness to others in this mysterious bestowal of a purely spiritual goodwill. Blessing is definitely good for the blesser as well as for the blessee.

Saints and angels are particularly good at blessings and they usually have radiantly good health and excellent postures. In contrast, the person who curses is traditionally pictured as screwed up and physically damaged by all that ill will.

People used to bless each other in daily greetings. "Goodbye", is still really "God be with you", and this is a fundamental blessing. It puts you right in the

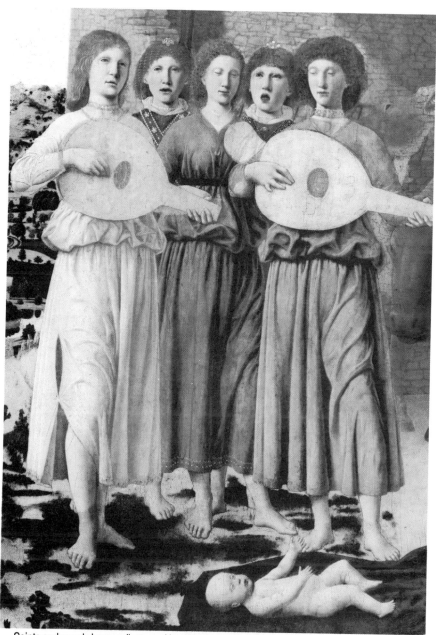

Saints and angels have radiant good health and excellent posture (*Pero Della Francesca: The Nativity – Detail; rep'roduced by courtesy of The Trustees, The National Gallery, London*)

centre of universal intelligence! Perhaps our forebears were more willing to invite God into each other's lives. We mostly now only allow ourselves the right to bless someone when they sneeze or perhaps if they do us a favour! Without becoming obsessive about this exercise for the spirit we could easily make a few more opportunities to bless one another, bringing a little invisible spiritual lubricant to the welfare of our bodies and minds.

A nice bonus from exercising in these various spiritual ways, is that we start to notice that we too are, in any case, loved, forgiven, appreciated and blest. We become aware that we are already surrounded by priceless gifts and blessed with fitness and natural healing.

Start sometimes at the S end when exercising your fitness team. Make it an S/M/B enterprise, for a refreshing change. If you are afraid you may be doing this for personal gain alone, expand your thinking. Guilt does not come into it. See the whole human network expanding just one small fraction, too, just because you chose to expand your fitness.

Modern scientific theory claims that when a butterfly moves its wings in one small location, the rest of the universe experiences and responds to that flutter. Be the butterfly! Create that positive flutter! Making new experiences is a human speciality, a gift that we owe to consciousness.

Body work, we all know, helps minds and spirits to flourish. Do some! Mental work brings intelligence and imagination to the way we use bodies and spirits. Use it! And some conscious gentle warm-ups, stretches, loosening up and toning exercises for our spirit will always act as a fillip for bodies and minds as well. Keep fitting them in!

EXERCISE SECTION 13

Feeling Better: The Basics of Emotional Tension Release

The Exercises

Emotional Awareness

The *feeling* side of our lives affects body, mind and spirit. Like the sensory information we use for balance and proprioception, feelings are a part of the way in which we can tell where and how we are. When we use them well we can handle the many challenging downward pulls in life that seem as ever present as gravity is for bodies. But our feelings can sometimes play tricks on us and some techniques for managing difficult ones can play a big part in our fitness, including our confidence and vital self valuing.

The exercises outlined for this very personal area are, again, with the aim of expanding awareness. Even one experimental exercise can make us more aware of the emotional pageant going on and help us to clear negative emotions out of the way and make way for better ones.

In the civilised world, although we value spontaneity, we don't always have to act upon every immediate feeling. The great step forward out of animal life into human consciousness lets us put a delay between *signal* and *response*, and making that pause is one of the most useful exercises we can do. Inside it, moment by moment, lies our only opportunity to make conscious choice and we can learn to make better choices. We can choose to fade out some self pity and unhappiness and introduce, perhaps little by little, experimentally, more positive responses.

When we can stand back from our emotions, they may clarify. We need not hide them so much from ourselves and others nor inflict the negative ones on those around us, so often. We can stop letting the painful ones dominate our lives for too long, undermining our well-being. We can focus more on the things that feel good, really are good and are going well.

Carl Rogers' work as a gifted and very aware counsellor, made plain the value of openness and authenticity in everybody's emotional life. He found in his therapeutic work, that when real feelings are acknowledged and not disguised, either by counsellor or client, real healing can take place. When he as counsellor hid his own feelings and reactions from the client, out of sympathy and (perhaps mistaken) kindness, he noticed that the therapy seemed hampered. But in a direct expression of his own feelings of the moment, when he might say, for example: "when you said that I felt you were trying to use or manipulate me", he found his client becoming more open and authentic in expressing his own feelings, too, and bringing out past events that could then be talked about openly.

The same is true in our ordinary relationships. We have some conventional behaviours and mutual respect to observe, of course, but severe suppression of feelings does not lead to healthy relationships between us. We are not therapists for each other exactly, but somehow, when we meet as authentic, emotionally aware people and can express what we are feeling without losing our positive regard for one another, there is a therapeutic aspect, a mutual healing opportunity all the time between people. We are able to give each other a climate in which each of us can heal old traumas and grow naturally and healthily. And we can also let this supportive process of openly acknowledging our own feelings work in our inner personal life.

Many of today's health and relationship problems are very closely linked. Troubles with either often stem directly from very early emotional upsets in which we first learned to hide the truth of how we felt. At a very vulnerable time we may have closed down in fear and self protection instead of staying open to and openly expressive of our feelings.

When we do suppress or hide a strong emotion our own energy has to be used to hold the lid on. Tension then develops, which affects the whole of us. We cannot tense up one part of ourselves without sending echoes right through the organism. Body, mind and spirit screw up together. But is there anything we can do now about feelings long past and our present reactions which often seem so strongly built in to our very nature?

I accept Carl Rogers' insight that we can sharpen our alertness and work to become much more aware of our feelings even at the time of having them. And I accept the wisdom that prevails in the therapy world today that there are practical things everyone can do to defuse even quite ancient emotional hang-ups without necessarily seeking individual professional counselling. I also recognise that if our troubles are very severe we do need specialist help. But most of us can safely bring recent or even quite long ago feelings into much sharper focus by some inner work of our own.

By looking at any of our upsetting emotions afresh we can usually remove little by little some of the strong negative charge that they may have had for many years. Then we are able to let go of them, or they may just leave of their own accord and we forget we were ever troubled by them.

Some Emotions Undermine Us

Feelings find their way into the nervous system of the body, just as thoughts and attitudes do. They are all part of the information the brain uses as it regulates whole body functioning. The good ones steadily generate good chemistry for us but the bad ones, even those from long ago, can undermine us insidiously. People who seem to be somehow apologetic in their posture, very domineering or repeatedly negative in the things they say about themselves, others and the world, almost certainly have old emotional patterns hidden away. It is then very valuable to work for some emotional release as well as directly on physical loosening up and toning exercises and posture. Many body work therapists agree that the emotional backlog is often the main obstacle when other apparently physical problems are failing to mend.

We are usually surprisingly reluctant to part with our negative emotions, either present ones, nagging at us right now, or those from long ago. We tend to treat our feelings as always sacrosanct and hang on to them tightly. They are important, of course, and very much ours, but we can too easily make the mistake of identifying them with our personal worth. We hate other people to hurt our feelings. Yet if those feelings are an exaggerated reaction, a throw back to unresolved experiences from long ago, we are doing the present hurting ourselves and need not blame the other person for triggering an old sensitive issue accidentally.

When we feel secure and confident we can easily shrug off a snub, for example, but if deeply anxious we may smart for years about it. With emotional maturity it should be possible to remain unhurt by many of the slings and arrows of daily living. When we are able to realise we have been doing the hurting ourselves, in an unconscious play back of old fears, we can grow up a little and learn to let go of it. We can spot the *I feel hurt* reaction as it comes in and accept it as a passing event. Instead of slamming into our defensive automatic responses, we could just yield to it momentarily, register that it happened, and then let it go.

We don't want to live in general mistrust of anybody's healthy feelings or of our own. The positive ones deserve to be savoured and enjoyed, but if a distorted and out-of-date negative pattern is there, probably locked up in nerve and muscle blockages, it would be nice to find ways to be rid of it.

Humans do not have to act from ancient instructions for ever. Our past does not have to determine our future. We can make better use of our rational mind and learn to notice first, and then resolve some of our emotional disturbances almost as soon as they arise.

The exercises of this chapter do not deny or belittle anybody's feelings. They are about looking more closely, reviewing where they arose, and then taking time to let some of them fade away or quietly evaporate. Afterwards, again as with the body work, it is good to acknowledge our progress and let the messages sink in. If we feel more at ease in the new emotional freedom we say so, to ourselves if not to others, and then we simply enjoy the new release.

Some of the emotional left overs we are better without can be a result of quite minor misjudgements or fears. An overheard remark or a rather thought-less rebuff can linger for a long time. Some may be remnants of very real past pains. To the infant, quite small incidents, not necessarily intended unkindly, will have seemed hugely threatening and frightening. Hidden away, these can still be triggered again and again and then colour quite different events. When a mere hint of a repeat situation threatens, the body/mind sees a resemblance to the earlier situation and we feel instant panic and threat automatically all over again. As the survival response switches on we recoil instantly mentally, ready for *fight or flight*, just as fast as taking our hand off a hot stove.

When the brain switches in this way its logical part cuts off and is temporarily lost to us, and this is the cooperation we want to restore. A strong emotional replay can paralyse our rational thinking. For a time we are run by the purely imaginary threat thrown up from the past. All our defences stiffen and the body stiffens too. Breathing becomes more shallow. Muscles become more tense. Our perceptions shrink and tighten, so that even vision and hearing partly close down. We can become aggressive, sulk or shrink into an all over avoidance mode just as we may once have done protectively as a child. We are obviously not in full command to make rational decisions if we have reacted in this way, yet we are often completely unaware that this automatic behaviour is going on.

If you doubt that this sort of reaction, into irrational levels of upset, could ever happen to you, just notice that it happens to almost everybody you know, and then wonder why you should be immune. It is natural and instructive, not nosy, to notice other people and be aware of their feelings. We are all useful mirrors to each other.

Curiosity about the feelings of others is one of the conscious mind's very useful awareness skills. We develop it quite early. Empathy and sympathy are important to humans. People who have not learned when they were infants to notice the feelings of others, are seriously handicapped, with autism the extreme example of such a lack. Even a partial inability to notice that other people have feelings, too, can lead to an insensitivity that shows up right through life. But if we sharpen and use our natural observation and curiosity we can come to accept that *having one's feelings hurt* does throw quite rational people, even you and me sometimes, into pre-programmed reactions that are very strong.

Some of our strong, quite automatic reactions may have been laid down even longer ago, not even in our personal history but in our shared evolutionary past, even in our genes. We can recognise some quite *farmyard* behaviours in each other at times. There are many primitive behaviour patterns we share with other species. But wherever they come from, once we notice that what is happening is automatic in a conditioned or programmed way, we can encourage the logical left brain to take a new detached look at the experience, and we then, at least, have an opportunity to change our response to it.

These exercises are simply about making that new look possible and opening up the possibility of freeing our emotions from past events, so that we can be authentic in our feelings now, and fully expressive of current joys and present sadnesses and open to others in theirs.

Releasing the Minus to Liberate the Plus: A Mini-Exercise

This is a very simple introductory exercise. It only takes a few minutes, so when familiar it can be fitted into small gaps of time. If we practise it, even occasionally, it alerts us to start to observe something in ourselves that we might not have noticed. Many of us hate any idea of self observation. But don't dismiss this exercise as idle navel-watching unless you are willing to ignore an important aspect of your holistic well-being. The reason we turn away from self searching is often a hidden fear of what we might find there. Be brave! The exercise takes much less time to do than to describe and is in no way dangerous.

Look first at how you are feeling now! If all is rosy and well, enjoy that fact and get new energy from it. Bring it more clearly into your awareness: "I feel well, that's nice!" Or "I feel brilliant!", "I feel wonderful!" But then see if you can waylay any small tension or negative feeling going on anywhere in the background of your mind. As with body tensions, if we think around the body, or in this case the emotions, we can often locate and let go of one that was not obvious before. If no present negative flutter comes to mind, go back a little in time. There will usually be some recent minor upset to work on. ("I felt such a fool yesterday!" for example.) If this search also fails then simply, for this exercise, imagine yourself feeling upset about anything at all.

You could choose being just mildly annoyed at your neighbour because her washing line or bonfire offends you. Or you could be feeling a pang of imagined inferiority to someone you have recently met. Take any negative flutter, like feeling snubbed, slighted, criticised or annoyed. Or take a memory of something stupid you once did in the not-too-distant past and now regret, or someone once letting you down. We carry a surprising number of these emotional ripples. Pick one.

Relax, breathe fully, close your eyes, and put your minor upset feelings into words. "I seem to hate Mrs. X. today", for example, or "I wish I hadn't made such a *faux pas* last week!" Your mind will try to run away, but you can chase it and hold it to its purpose. You can be in charge of this team member. Only when we stand back from our feelings can we act completely rationally. Even while trying to stand back you will almost certainly want to justify and perhaps strengthen the feelings, ("but Mrs. X. really is terrible!"). Just push past these negative thoughts, too, because they are all probably also reactions that just arose automatically.

A first initiative could be to recruit your spirit and practise some of the positive exercises of appreciation, love and forgiveness. Try one now! In the *bad neighbour* example, try forgiving her for being herself, and yourself for being as you are, and all neighbourly problems everywhere, big and small, for being as they are. This may be all that is needed! But then widen the field, right away from the personal aspect. Take a look at relationships all around the human race. None of us was born with a guarantee that everything would work out perfectly to suit our every wish through the whole of our life.

Irritations just like these have always been common at community and even international levels. Even in the early Greek city states, so proud of their rational and civilised culture, it was often the nearest neighbour state to whom they felt most hostile. It was quite usual for alliances and treaties to be made with the states beyond the neighbour, rather than with the one next door who seemed much more threatening and difficult.

A neighbourly threat is very close to us and we have automatic wariness about it. Modern neighbours and neighbour nations, still squabble today as they have for hundreds of years. Somehow we need to make an extra psychological effort if we are to break out of the whole primitive pattern involved in suspicion between neighbours and find ways of being truly neighbourly with them.

If your feelings are still strongly negative, even after that objective widening of the view, start to look for specific bodily reactions. Some of the feelings will be there as tightness in hands, jaw, back or elsewhere in the body. If you can locate or even imagine such a localised tension, sit or lie in one of the relaxation postures and get down to some creative visualisation to be rid of it. Hold your fingertips lightly on the bones of the upper forehead for a minute or two. Imagine that you are drawing out the old reactions that triggered this annoyance and are giving your brain freedom to be actively positive again.

I have taken chest tightness in my example because tightness of the ribs and breathing almost always accompanies held back emotions. But you could work on the hands, jaw, forehead or feet if you detect particular tension in these.

Act out a fanciful mental visualisation in full colourful detail in which you give the tension some definite shape, size and reality. It might feel like an iron hard or stony obstruction sitting in your chest. Then set out to open up the tight area. You could visualise a surgical operation, for example, and remove a whole box full of weights or pebbles! Or pour in some magic fluid that can first dissolve and then swoosh all the heavy material away.

You can direct your breath to expand and nourish the areas involved. Imagine breathing oxygen right into the tight places. You can involve your own spiritual guides or people who inspire you, and ask them in imagination to remove the blocks. Watch them lift out the culprit material and carry it bodily away.

Take a few minutes to do some imaginative inner operation of this sort. It can be quite light hearted, but you will feel a lessening of tension and a new lightness. You might even laugh about how unnecessary all the fuss was. You can say goodbye to your tensions as they disperse or dissolve or are visibly carted away and can experience real relief and freedom.

To sum up this basic process, for general, practical use:

☐ Pause to see what is happening

☐ Bring some generosity of spirit to the scene

☐ Widen your viewpoint from personal to bigger relationships

☐ Play-act a removal of the problem, in very vivid terms

☐ Relax. Declare the emotional stress to have faded or gone

☐ Acknowledge the freedom and lightness that follow.

The second exercise takes longer and goes more deeply. If you know that you have excessively cruel experiences in your past, this more deeply searching process is not for you. Don't try to unravel experiences that have been unnaturally cruel or severe without an experienced person to support you. Stay, instead, with the mini-exercise above, for minor troubles, and become proficient with that one. If reading my imagined examples leads you to want to work on distressing long ago past traumas, find a skilled counsellor to guide and stay with you as you go through unnaturally painful early memories.

Digging Deeper

Our personal history has much in common with the history of our race. Each inevitably has lots of mistakes and rubbish in it. The personal rubbish can include old feelings of resentment, guilts, fears and pains and probably feelings of rejection and inadequacy, too. All that has been good in our past has been incorporated into the positive qualities of our life now, and this is the stuff we grow by. But it is vital to keep dissolving away all lingering legacies of the bad, even from very long ago, because these cause continuing pain and simply hold us back from growth and health. They make it hard for us to keep up the positive and outward momentum, even in the basic everyday body work, that we need in the *direction of plus*.

Many workers in bodily fitness and movement education, not just doctors and counsellors, have noticed that a lot of health problems have their origin in emotional problems. These may, of course, sometimes be from recent hurts, such as a divorce or bereavement, but even our response to recent major events can have roots that go deeply into the past.

F.M. Alexander early in the 20th century was one of the first to make these links between present physical problems, and past emotional ones. Wilhelm Reich was another. Many others have either followed in their footsteps or independently worked in body work or counselling to help to clear away the emotional backlog and to heal through similar insights.

Janet Goodrich today, in her work of Natural Vision Improvement, stresses this problem of emotional tensions as one of the most important factors in defective vision. Patsy Rodenburg working with the voice acknowledges its importance to use of the breath in singing and acting. Almost all *alternative* therapists as well as teachers of vision, hearing or voice improvement are today acknowledging this fact. Their individual approach may have an emphasis towards spiritual, psychological or body work according to their special interest, but freeing the emotional backlog is very often an essential part of the therapy or healing process for each of these areas.

The following longer exercise for emotional release is like a home therapy session. It takes time, but then we cannot just *wish* our emotional rubbish away. Don't do this exercise at once, but read it through and think about giving time to it when you next feel unhappy or cross.

If you are hesitant, notice that emotional stresses are absolutely normal and quite as common as physical knocks. The resilient human race has always suffered from both varieties and we can see them as similarly healable. Don't feel ashamed about having emotional stuff to work on. No one avoids these. Treat your past hurts rather matter-of-factly, as well as sympathetically, perhaps as you would a child's hurt knee. It is a domestic *kiss it better* treatment, not an emergency ward drama!

The body/mind is being asked to bring its powerful healing resources into the emotional as well as the bodily arena. We shall be using a "there, there, that wasn't so bad really!" in the emotional scene just as we cheerfully do for physical knocks for a child. It need not be heavy going.

Next time you feel strongly enraged, upset or just rather miserable, pause to notice that feeling and give yourself time to examine it more deeply. Make a deliberate pause as an exercise. Show yourself that such a pause is possible. Go somewhere quiet and make a break in all other activities for several minutes. If you can throw any light at all on this strong surge of negative emotion it can help you to become freer of many other similar episodes. A whole string of them can unravel. You can become free to enjoy all the positive emotions much more fully. Without making such a break and deliberately choosing to try something different, you may be stuck with repetitions of this one, over and over again.

The essence of this deeper exercise is not simply to notice or wallow in the flurry of today's feelings, but to go far back in time. We see if we can remember any early incident when we have felt similar feelings. Then we look earlier still and keep going until we reach the earliest experience we can remember, of loss, rejection, irrational rage or whatever it is. Then we stay with the memory of that early emotion and have a close look at the experience that led to it. It is the unfinished business of scenes which we have brushed aside as misunderstood or too painful at the time, that stays trapped.

There is a *sandwich* shape to this exercise. At the beginning and end we need detachment and logical appraisal. But right in the middle we let go of those and immerse ourselves in an experiential re-play of our past, very strong feelings. Afterwards we are able to accept the whole experience quite rationally and let it retreat benignly into the neutral past.

The hardest part may be in resisting the temptation to brush the emotion aside. But running away from our hang-ups does not set us free. We need to be brave, curious and willing to look deeply. We have to go in imagination right into the early scene as if it were now and notice how acutely unhappy we felt then.

Be fully there. Face that situation head on. Re-live it. Soon you will be recognising that, although you had every reason to feel upset when that happened, it is over now and you are able to let it go.

The exercise is described very fully because we do need to immerse ourselves in all its detail before a new release can be found. The example that follows is a very slight one, to illustrate the main points. Use it only as a guide. It is in the first person and present tense. We need to use "I" to be totally in the scene we recall. Your own exercise afterwards can follow this pattern whatever past incident you choose to replay.

I have found myself feeling very miserable for no apparent reason. So I have stopped everything else to enquire within. I have overcome my reluctance to look at the feelings that are going on in me and I am searching my recent memory. Then I discover that this surprisingly strong emotion has not come *out of the blue* but has been triggered by a particular event this morning.

I had suggested a nice outing with my husband, and he had dismissed the idea because he had too many other commitments. I thought he had been rather abrupt but I had accepted his decision cheerfully. It made obvious sense. But now I seem to have a nagging misery encroaching on everything else. Life seems unfair on a broad front. That apparently trivial incident must have had quite a big emotional charge.

So I start my detective work! Can I recall ever feeling unhappy in this way before? Then other memories begin to appear. Yes! I realise that I have felt like this quite often in similar or even quite different circumstances. There was an incident only last week when I felt slighted by an acquaintance and I was cross and unhappy all day. I recall similar feelings a few weeks ago. And more last Christmas. And yes, I realise that such feelings have often recurred over many years. This begins to look interesting! A recurrent pattern has emerged.

By stopping to sort out where my present mood began, I have detached myself from it a little and the left brain is curious and engaged.

Going earlier still, looking for the very earliest feeling I can remember of being apparently rejected like this, I find I can go right back to a memory of feeling extremely sorry for myself as a child of about three. A brother or sister has refused to play with me, and suddenly I feel very small. I feel unwanted, frighteningly unloved and totally wretched.

Take a good look at your own earliest scene. It may be quite a trivial incident, but the fact that it has popped up to be remembered means it is worth looking at now. If it was a time when you were severely punished or hurt, try not to over-dramatise it as you review it, but take time to be there, in the present moment as it was then, and re-live it, recalling all the surroundings as well, not just the way you felt.

"I am in the garden at home, quite early after breakfast. I am three. I am alone. I am wearing a blue flowery cotton dress and white knickers that my mother made. It is summer. I am in the sand pit with a wooden spoon, a tin mug and a small red and yellow tin bucket with a scratched picture of starfishes and seaweed on it. There are some wet leaves and stones in the sand too, and I am starting to make sand pies."

Keep on exploring the detail of what is there. The sand is warm and dry on top, damp and cold underneath. The garden wall is old and made of chalky crumbly reddish bricks. It feels warm from the sun. I can smell rhubarb and compost in the vegetable plot and nearby I can see cabbage leaves nearly as big as me. I am sitting still, all alone, hanging my head. I am feeling bereft because I just asked my brother to play with me and he said I was silly. Then he went away to play with my bigger sister indoors. I don't feel silly. I feel entirely good. Surely he must want to play with me most.

Use all the visual detail you can recall, and include sounds and scents too, everything that brings back the reality of that event. Even that remembered incident may not be your very first encounter with the devastating feelings of childhood rejection, so don't give this one an exaggerated importance. Just keep on re-living your feelings, using all your senses. See and feel the sand and taste your hot tears and intensify all the feelings you had then.

After living in the whole memory for several minutes, seeing and hearing more and more detail, put those early unhappy feelings into words. Speak them aloud: "I feel terrible!", "I'm shrinking and tight all over", "It feels like the end of the world!" "I love my brother so much and I thought he loved me too!", "Nobody loves me!" Sit there, bowed and forlorn in the morning sunshine in the sand pit you remember, and express in words now, all the despair and anguish you felt long ago as a three year old.

It is possible you may cry again, because re-living our early feelings taps into that inner river of tears. Let tears come if they want, but don't make a big orgy of crying. Keep your left brain available, even while your right brain takes this journey into the strong emotions of the past. It is while you are expressing the situation in words, a left brain involvement, that you will start to bring a new balance to your perceptions. You will begin to see those words having relevance for you today. "I thought he loved me." "Perhaps nobody loves me!" "I feel small and hopeless!" "Perhaps I have to be bigger and cleverer to be loveable." "Things ought to be better than this!"

After putting these deep early anxieties into words and getting back to some of the unhappiness of a three year old, you may begin to feel some relaxing of the upsetting emotions. They feel less urgent. You emerge a little. You feel clearer and more detached from them, perhaps a little more grown up, even beginning to be bored with them! You may even start to notice more of the good things about that sunny morning. You feel lighter and less hunched. You look around you. You expand your body and breathing. "Perhaps I can still play with the sand! I like these buckets and spades, and the sun is nice and warm. Someone will come and play with me soon."

Bathe the whole scene imaginatively in more positive images of light and love and a dawning joy. Begin to play again, to laugh again and feel sand trickling through your fingers and all the wonderful pleasures of summer childhood mornings. You have started to let go of the deeply hurt feelings of that remote but important small incident. At the time there was no one to help you past the anguish or support you in that little instance of learning.

Gradually bring your grown up wisdom to the same scene. Your adult self can see now that it was completely natural to have been so unhappy at that time. Children unavoidably sometimes are. They are very vulnerable at three years old. Misery does happen to human beings and always has, and very few people escape its pangs. It feels terrible at the time of experiencing it. It is especially intense for the small infant with slender resources, so little experience and such dependence on those around her. But the pain need not go on for ever. This incident belongs in the long distant past and can fade away now.

Your logical mind is re-entering. You are recognising that although infants may go through heart breaking troubles it is possible to recover completely and emerge emotionally strong and happy again. It will extend that insight to other events as well and you will feel stronger. It is an opportunity for new growth in self support and more acceptance of other people too and their separate wants and needs. If a kind parent had been there with a loving hug at the time, the whole episode would have melted into the past then and there and left no scar.

You are doing your own hugging now, from your mature self to yourself as a child. You are the only person now who can do that fully for you. You accept the child you were, completely, and all of the experiences and feelings s/he ever had, and will no longer need to keep replaying that tape or having to handle those churned up feelings. If they do come round again you will let them go by more quickly and easily.

In that deliberately relived experience, which is more effective than any analytical thoughts about your upset, you recognise experientially how vulnerable you were then. But because you are grown up and intelligent now, you can also feel the child's growing strength and your own adult strength. Pathways in the brain that were partially paralysed by that early stress have healed and become active again. You find an interesting responsibility to take charge of your own feelings and create new happiness for yourself.

As you shift your attention deliberately to positive things, remember some of life's many happier truths. Think about people then and now whom you love and who love you too. Feel blessed and secure in the love of your parents, family and many friends. Feel happiness returning to the child you were and imagine her going back to contented play, the emotional hurt healing over.

For a farewell flourish to this exercise, now embark on painting the physical details extravagantly brightly. See the sun shining higher and still more brilliantly in the sky, and the sky more wonderfully blue. See flowers blooming and hear the birds singing and the church bells ringing joyfully. See your brothers and sisters coming out to play again, full of fun and with new games to share with you. Say aloud: "Yes! All of that and more can and did happen to me, as it does to everybody else. I felt devastated then, yet all is still well! I am loved and I'm lovable and loving too and the world is beautiful. I can see that just at that time he didn't feel like playing in the sand. I'm happy with that. People do have lots of interests and friends and so do I. The world has certainly not come to an end, it is full of sunshine and promise."

Turn your attention to whomever was involved for you in that early scene, as you let it go, and use your imagination to surround these persons with light and love or showers of rose petals or any other fancy right brain symbols of forgiveness and joy that you like to invent! Forgive them with all your heart, even if they may have died long ago. Those involved in our past hurts inevitably share our human limitations. You can see them now as also loving and good, getting on with their own life in their own way, doing the best they can. Give them your blessing and wish them well.

Before leaving this exercise, go from your particular example out into the general scheme of things. Widen the view. Think a little more about how, in the whole of human experience, not one of us has a totally peaceful history or can expect everything to go our way all the time. Yet, from small or large mishaps we are able to heal and pick up the pieces to put life together again and continue to grow and to generate good feelings. We still have our unique feelings and emotional needs but we can free ourselves to find healthy ways to express those feelings and meet those needs.

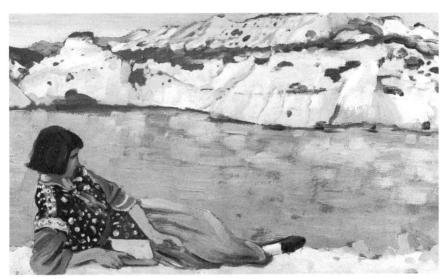

Sometimes, just being in the world and alive to its beauty and its mystery is all that we need
(The Blue Pool by Augustus John; reproduced by permission of City of Aberdeen Art Gallery & Museums Collection)

Courage and Healing

This is an existential matter, of course, not just a personal one. It takes courage for anyone to pick him or herself up, but human beings are courageous. We are made that way. We are part of a natural world in which courage and healing are essential ingredients. If it were not so, life would have given up long ago.

Old scars can heal well, and the process is well on the way for you after this exercise. Some delayed growth has happened. You have stepped forward into a bigger adulthood that puts you more firmly in the picture as an important provider of love and healing in your own life and in that of others, too. You will start to feel less at the mercy of your perceived needs; more able to give love as well as to receive it. You are more secure now and can exercise your own strength. You can feel hurt for a shorter time whenever that crippling reaction comes in.

The past is healing over, you are very strong in the present, and the future is opening up brighter and better prospects. You are no longer such a victim of your own feelings or other people's whims but shape your actions firmly. You meet others in your strength now, not from those painful flashbacks into earlier vulnerability.

You may only want to use this deeply searching exercise very occasionally, perhaps only once. But each time we pause to look at our negative emotions objectively and release an old or new emotional hurt, we become more aware of the irrational aspect of storing any of them. We do not have to become *thick skinned,* but we can become more generously tolerant and much less ready to take offence, more open and clear in our feelings, and able to express them and move along. Our faculties remain healthily available instead of throttled, and we become more able to cope with today's events in today's best and healthiest way.

But that is enough of exercises for now! There is a lot of life to be living without exercising all the time! Sometimes just being in the world and alive to its beauty and its mystery is all that we need. But with practice and understanding we become more and more efficient in our use of this and any of the B/M/S exercises, especially if we see them as part of a bigger picture of our fitness in the setting of our expanding B/M/S awareness.

We can use small scraps of or cracks in our timetables purposefully and well, physically or emotionally, to loosen up or stretch or release old tensions and create new positive goals. We can fit small exercises between the many other creative and productive pursuits we are involved in. And from time to time we can get down to a longer topping up session, treating ourselves to some in-depth work.

Be patient! You have all of the rest of your life to work with these ideas. And the exercises themselves simply continue to teach you, if you do them thoroughly, as you will see.

After any consciously positive exercise, even the tiny ones, we go back to our other tasks much better equipped. We feel more balanced in our posture and attitudes, more centred and strong, more mentally alert and altogether more alive. We balance the apparent opposites of our self caring and our ability to give to others, we get better at managing these seeming contradictions.

That should all make the world just a wee bit better for everybody!

Bibliography

Fitness, Exercise and Movement

Christopher Connolly & Hetty Einzig, *The Fitness Jungle*, Century.

Sue Luby & Richard St Onge, *Bodysense*, Faber and Faber Inc., 50 Corn Street, Winchester, MA 01890, USA.

The Alexander Technique

F.M. Alexander, *The Use of the Self*, Victor Gollancz.

Wilfred Barlow, *The Alexander Principle*, Victor Gollancz.

Michael Gelb, *Body Learning*, Aurum Press.

Judith Leibowitz & Bill Connington, *The Alexander Technique*, Souvenir Press.

Glen Park, *The Art of Changing*, Ashgrove.

Body Awareness

Ken Dychtwald, *Bodymind*, Wildwood House, London.

Moshe Feldenkraus, *Awareness Through Movement*, Penguin.

Alexander Lowen, *Bioenergetics*, Penguin.

John Syer and Christopher Connolly, *Sporting Body, Sporting Mind*, C.U.P.

Mind Brain and Vision

Tony Buzan, *Make the Most of Your Mind*, Pan.

Janet Goodrich, *Natural Vision Improvement*, Viking O'Neil.

Ronald Shone, *Creative Visualization*, Thorsons.

Evolutionary Perspectives

Bernard Campbell, *Human Evolution*, Heinemann Educational Books Ltd.

Nicholas Humphrey, *Consciousness Regained*, O.U.P.

Jean Liedloff, *The Continuum Concept*, Penguin.

Health and Self Healing
Louise L. Hay, *You Can Heal Your Life,* Eden Grove Editions.
C. Norman Shealy & Caroline Myss, *The Creation of Health,* Stillpoint.

Life Energy
Peter Schellenbaum, *The Wound of the Unloved,* Element Books.

The Body and Movement
Lucy Lidell, *The Sensual Body,* Unwin.

Inner Game
Timothy Gallwey, *The Inner Game of Tennis,* Jonathan Cape.
Timothy Gallwey & Bob Kriegel, *Inner Skiing,* Bantam.

Tai Chi
Cheng Man-ch'ing, *T'ai Chi Ch'uan,* North Atlanta Books, California.
Lawrence Galante, *Tai Chi The Supreme Ultimate,* Samuel Weiser, Miami.
Bob Klein, *Movements and Magic,* Newcastle Publishing, California.

Voice and Music
Patsy Rodenburg, *The Right to Speak,* Methuen Drama.
Anthony Storr, *Music & the Mind,* Harper Collins.

Zen
Shunryu Suzuki, *Zen Mind, Beginner's Mind,* Weatherhill.

Acknowledgements

There are many individual teachers and others I would like to thank for showing me things that are important for bodies minds and spirits, and giving me ideas that have been used in this book. Each has illuminated different aspects of exercise and fitness for me, and my own teaching in the field of movement education has drawn from all of them. I have also learnt a great deal from the many men and women who have worked with me in my classes. Thank you to you all.

I am saying more general thankyous here as if to the several separate areas from which I have learnt, rather than the many individuals. This is partly to declare the main influences in my work but is also intended as acknowledgment of those wonderful individuals who taught me. In nearly every case, a teacher in one field recommended the particular work and skills of another. It was in looking for common principles to all that worked best for me, that I developed my own approach to exercise.

I have often been asked how I came to teach an exercise programme after being a maths teacher (left brain work), then a potter (more right brain activated), and then a grandmother of 10 (multi-skilled role!). The wide range of these acknowledgments shows why it is so hard to answer that in only a few words. I was athletic when young and always fascinated by movement, sports and body work. My interest even then ranged from ancient to modern cultures and from East to West, but a wartime choice of career turned me to other fields. When comparatively late in life I decided I wanted to carry this life long interest into teaching, it has been quite a challenge to create a practical everyday programme that could use so many sources yet be useful and not confusing to a general fitness seeker. I was keen to help to switch our culture away from its creeping measure of bodily neglect. I used every idea that had worked for me.

The Alexander Technique

In F.M. Alexander's work, I first learnt the importance of length and of body awareness. I could begin to notice that bodies operate as a whole and the body/mind also operates as an entity. I had read all Alexander's books very early in my life but his lessons were an experiential breakthrough into body awareness for me. Those lessons have spread over many years, via gifted and generous teachers and they still open up new freedoms for me.

Tai Chi Chuan

In the gentle oriental martial art of Tai Chi, recommended to me by my first Alexander teacher, I grew to enjoy feeling my feet firmly on the ground and the top of my head directed right up to the sky, with a nice feeling of extension between these opposites. Tai Chi also gave me the message that it is important to face squarely and practically in the direction one wishes to pursue.

The ancient philosophical teachings of Tai Chi speak of the mind directing the body. This gave me the courage, when I started to teach, to speak to bodies and minds as if they belonged together. Oriental teachers had no doubts about this. Tai Chi exercises also assume that the *chi*, or life spirit flows in the individual as well as right through the universe, and that loosening up exercises free us from blockages that hamper the chi, and encourage its health-giving flow. That seemed a nice image to adopt. I rarely miss my daily Tai Chi practice.

All of the martial arts have taken inspiration from the beauty and efficiency of the movements of animals and birds. They incorporate imitations of these into many of their exercises. I had always liked to fit myself into the evolutionary picture and I began to see much useful information in animal movement and our evolutionary inheritance. Wild life films and visits to large zoos where freedom is respected, can tell us a lot about the missing element of wide ranging movement in modern human lives.

Aston Fitness

The Eastern influence in my training was complemented by wisdom from the West, from up-to-the-minute California. Under Judith Aston's tuition, in courses she gave in London first, and then at her school in the USA, I said goodbye to any residual imagining that bodies might ever benefit from regimental or masochistic training. (Animals never *march* except in circuses). Perhaps soldiers need symmetry and abrupt movements, but for most of us these can do lasting harm.

Judith Aston's work has a strong forward-directedness which fitted with and strengthened my own inclination towards all the positives of life, as did her emphasis on having good images towards which to work. And it was Judith's very definite eschewal of imposed symmetry and jarring that led me to think further about the evolutionary and mechanical factors involved, and the conditions and movements that bodies actually expect and need.

Natural Vision

It was a long time ago that I first heard of W.H. Bates' method for better eyesight. My father had had lessons with a Bates practitioner and it impressed me that he had given up his reading glasses quite late in life. I learnt then that movement and simple exercises bring benefits to eyes. Somewhat later I had a few lessons with a teacher, almost 90 years old then, who had trained with W.H. Bates and still had wonderfully good eyesight. Later still, in courses in England and then in Australia, I studied with Dr Janet Goodrich whose world renowned work has built on that of Dr Bates.

As with Judith Aston's work, Janet Goodrich's totally positive and vision-ary directedness left its mark on my fitness and exercise teaching and my life. Influences on her own research included her 10 years of practice as a Reichian therapist before devoting all her work to Natural Vision. Wilhelm Reich's teaching about body armouring and the damage done by stored emotional stresses was carried into her understanding of common defects in vision.

The Natural Vision Improvement teaching and philosophy includes freeing up the brain with movement and relaxation, freeing neck and facial tensions, and stimulating coordination with exercises, all practices which benefit much more than our vision. No exercise plan of mine seemed complete after that without some *cross-crawl* or its variations, and some massage to complement neck exercises.

Janet Goodrich also pointed out, almost as an aside, that human generosity contributes to human wellbeing, and that our imagination can be a health asset, too. I found that in sorting out for this book the exercises that mattered to me, I wanted to include some easy exercises for imaginations and generous spirits as well.

The Inner Game

Timothy Gallwey's books first, and then Inner Game skiing holidays more practically, brought home to me the need to let go of mental and bodily tensions together, when learning a physical skill. My skiing improved in leaps and bounds! I managed, at last, to leave my critical faculty out of the picture and could throw myself into the sheer enjoyment of playing with new experiences on skis.

Moshe Feldenkrais's Teaching

I have had only a little experience from direct teaching of the Feldenkrais Method, but this was liberating. The slowing down of movement and the focusing of attention on tiny parts of a movement were akin to the Tai Chi and Alexander work, awakening muscles that had been almost asleep. It was also a revelation to notice how the whole body organises itself for even a small movement, and can release many restraints if we allow and encourage this all over involvement.

The World of Arts, Music and, especially, Crafts

My pottery and calligraphy teachers and many craftsmen colleagues and friends have been equally inspiring, although *exercise* in these areas may seem to be very different. They gave me much more than manual dexterity and practical know-how, necessary as those are. They showed me in their own work how human creativity and self expression always involve very sensitive physical movements, and that they can flow from fingertips, brush, pen, voice or via loom, chisels or musical instruments, as if channels were open right through the body, mind and spirit.

Few people take a physical skill to the stage where the spirit shines brightly through, but when it happens, that openness, connectedness and inspiring integrity are always there. Average mortals like myself can then use that example for a little extension in their own lives, not just with the management of a potter's wheel or penman's quill.

The World of Science

My school and university training, marriage, reading and many friendships keep the down-to-earth nature of scientific enquiry important to me. I like the rational mind and appreciate working within the laws of the physical universe. I admire the integrity of scientists and their amazing dedication and work, whether in physics, medicine, physiology or any other field.

But scientists don't always have definitive answers, or claim them, and they necessarily limit their enquiries to the world of the measurable and quantifiable. They are also always searching and learning like the rest of us and can change their minds every decade and properly do so, if new discoveries disallow earlier theories.

So along with the training I received in science, I break out at the edges, perhaps unscientifically, and allow my own imagination and a few miracles to have a place in my universe. A natural world that has healing, growth and metamorphosis and also consciousness and an inner desire for improvement built into it, needs more than weighing, measuring and dissecting to give us pictures to live by.

Beliefs are less important to me than images that inspire, and I expect that the science world has played its part in that reluctance to subscribe to one creed. When I write about the human spirit I have no hot line to a particular manifestation of spirit, just a lot of pleasure in mystery, some fun with imagination, and a great respect for humanity.

Putting it All Together

I acknowledge my teachers in all these special fields with my sincere thanks. And now, can a non-specialist presume to recommend a general approach to exercise for average human beings? I have tried to do this. I am supremely average myself and I have chosen, borrowed and invented exercises that have worked miracles for me. My distillation of what matters and what works, and all errors and omissions in it, are my own.

Index